7 Tesla MRI

Editor

MENG LAW

MAGNETIC RESONANCE IMAGING CLINICS OF NORTH AMERICA

www.mri.theclinics.com

Consulting Editors
SURESH K. MUKHERJI
LYNNE S. STEINBACH

February 2021 • Volume 29 • Number 1

ELSEVIER

1600 John F. Kennedy Boulevard • Suite 1800 • Philadelphia, Pennsylvania, 19103-2899

http://www.mri.theclinics.com

MRI CLINICS OF NORTH AMERICA Volume 29, Number 1
February 2021 ISSN 1064-9689, ISBN 13: 978-0-323-75604-4

Editor: John Vassallo (j.vassallo@elsevier.com)
Developmental Editor: Kristen Helm

Magnetic Resonance Imaging Clinics of North America (ISSN 1064-9689) is published quarterly by Elsevier Inc., 360 Park Avenue South, New York, NY 10010-1710. Months of issue are February, May, August, and November. Business and Editorial Offices: 1600 John F. Kennedy Blvd., Ste. 1800, Philadelphia, PA 19103-2899. Customer Service Office: 3251 Riverport Lane, Maryland Heights, MO 63043. Periodicals postage paid at New York, NY and additional mailing offices. Subscription prices are $404.00 per year (domestic individuals), $1037.00 per year (domestic institutions), $100.00 per year (domestic students/residents), $450.00 per year (Canadian individuals), $1063.00 per year (Canadian institutions), $567.00 per year (international individuals), $1063.00 per year (international institutions), $100.00 per year (Canadian students/residents), and $275.00 per year (international students/residents). International air speed delivery is included in all *Clinics* subscription prices. All prices are subject to change without notice. **POSTMASTER:** Send address changes to *Magnetic Resonance Imaging Clinics*, Elsevier Health Sciences Division, Subscription Customer Service, 3251 Riverport Lane, Maryland Heights, MO 63043. Customer Service (orders, claims, online, change of address): Elsevier Health Sciences Division, Subscription **Customer Service, 3251 Riverport Lane, Maryland Heights, MO 63043. Tel:1-800-654-2452 (U.S. and Canada); 314-447-8871 (outside U.S. and Canada). Fax: 314-447-8029. E-mail: journalscustomerservice-usa@elsevier.com (for print support); journalsonlinesupport-usa@elsevier.com (for online support)**.

Reprints. For copies of 100 or more of articles in this publication, please contact the Commercial Reprints Department, Elsevier Inc., 360 Park Avenue South, New York, NY 10010-1710. Tel.: 212-633-3874; Fax: 212-633-3820; E-mail: reprints@elsevier.com.

Magnetic Resonance Imaging Clinics of North America is covered in the *RSNA Index of Imaging Literature, MEDLINE/PubMed (Index Medicus),* and *EMBASE/Excerpta Medica.*

Contributors

CONSULTING EDITORS

SURESH K. MUKHERJI, MD, MBA, FACR
Clinical Professor, Marian University, Director of Head and Neck Radiology, ProScan Imaging, Regional Medical Director, Envision Physician Services, Carmel, Indiana, USA

LYNNE S. STEINBACH, MD, FACR
Emeritus Professor of Radiology on Full Recall, Department of Radiology and Biomedical Imaging, University of California, San Francisco, San Francisco, California, USA

EDITOR

MENG LAW, MBBS, FRANZCR, MD, FASFNR
Meng Law Chair and Program Director of Radiology and Nuclear Medicine, Alfred Health, Professor of Radiology, Monash University, Department of Electrical and Computer Systems Engineering, Monash University, Department of Neuroscience, Monash School of Medicine, Nursing and Health Sciences, Director iBRAIN–Integrated Biomedical Research in Artificial Intelligence and Neuroimaging, Monash University, Melbourne, Victoria, Australia; Professor of Neurological Surgery, Keck School of Medicine, University of Southern California, Professor Biomedical Engineering, Viterbi School of Engineering, University of Southern California, Los Angeles, California, USA

AUTHORS

GREGOR ADRIANY, PhD
Center for Magnetic Resonance Research (CMRR), University of Minnesota, Minneapolis, Minnesota, USA

EDWARD J. AUERBACH, PhD
Center for Magnetic Resonance Research (CMRR), University of Minnesota, Minneapolis, Minnesota, USA

PRITI BALCHANDANI, PhD
Associate Professor, Associate Director, Biomedical Engineering and Imaging Institute, Icahn School of Medicine at Mount Sinai, New York, New York, USA

GIUSEPPE BARISANO, MD
Neurosurgeon and PhD Candidate, Neuroscience Graduate Program, University of Southern California, Los Angeles, California, USA

BANG V. BUI, PhD
Associate Professor, C/O Department of Optometry and Vision Sciences, Department of Optometry and Vision Sciences, The University of Melbourne, Parkville, Victoria, Australia

GREGORY CHANG, MD
Associate Professor, Section Chief of Musculoskeletal Imaging, Department of Radiology, NYU Langone Health, Bernard and Irene Schwartz Center for Biomedical Imaging, New York, New York, USA

JON O. CLEARY, MD, PhD
Specialist Registrar in Clinical Radiology, Department of Radiology, Guy's and St. Thomas' NHS Foundation Trust, London, United Kingdom; The Melbourne Brain Centre Imaging Unit, Department of Radiology, The University of Melbourne, Parkville, Victoria, Australia

RACHEL M. CUSTER, MS
Project Assistant, Laboratory of Neuro Imaging, Stevens Neuroimaging and Informatics Institute, Keck School of Medicine of USC, University of Southern California, Los Angeles, California, USA

BRADLEY N. DELMAN, MD, MS
Associate Professor of Diagnostic, Molecular and Interventional Radiology, Icahn School of Medicine at Mount Sinai, New York, New York, USA

PHILLIP DiGIACOMO, MS
Graduate Student, Department of Bioengineering, Stanford University, Lucas Center for Imaging, Stanford, California, USA

JUTTA M. ELLERMANN, MD, PhD
Center for Magnetic Resonance Research (CMRR), University of Minnesota, Minneapolis, Minnesota, USA

ARCAN ERTÜRK, PhD
Center for Magnetic Resonance Research (CMRR), University of Minnesota, Minneapolis, Minnesota, USA

REBECCA K. GLARIN, PGDipMRI
MRI Supervisor, The Melbourne Brain Centre Imaging Unit, Department of Medicine and Radiology, The University of Melbourne, Department of Radiology, Royal Melbourne Hospital, Parkville, Victoria, Australia

ANDREA GRANT, ScD
Center for Magnetic Resonance Research (CMRR), University of Minnesota, Minneapolis, Minnesota, USA

XIAOXUAN HE, ME
Center for Magnetic Resonance Research (CMRR), University of Minnesota, Minneapolis, Minnesota, USA

STEPHEN E. JONES, MD, PhD
Vice-Chairman for Research and Academic Affairs, Section of Neuroradiology, Imaging Institute, Cleveland Clinic, Cleveland, Ohio, USA

SCOTT C. KOLBE, PhD
Department of Neuroscience, Central Clinical School, Monash University, Prahran, Victoria, Australia

RUSSELL LAGORE, ME
Center for Magnetic Resonance Research (CMRR), University of Minnesota, Minneapolis, Minnesota, USA

MENG LAW, MBBS, FRANZCR, MD, FASFNR
Meng Law Chair and Program Director of Radiology and Nuclear Medicine, Alfred Health, Professor of Radiology, Monash University, Department of Electrical and Computer Systems Engineering, Monash University, Department of Neuroscience, Monash School of Medicine, Nursing and Health Sciences, Director iBRAIN-Integrated Biomedical Research in Artificial Intelligence and Neuroimaging, Monash University, Melbourne, Victoria, Australia; Professor of Neurological Surgery, Keck School of Medicine, University of Southern California, Professor Biomedical Engineering, Viterbi School of Engineering, University of Southern California, Los Angeles, California, USA

JONATHAN LEE, MD
Staff Neuroradiologist, Section of Neuroradiology, Imaging Institute, Cleveland Clinic, Cleveland, Ohio, USA

JANINE M. LUPO, PhD
Department of Radiology and Biomedical Imaging, University of California, San Francisco, San Francisco, California, USA

SAMANTHA J. MA, PhD
Laboratory of FMRI Technology (LOFT), USC Mark & Mary Stevens Neuroimaging and Informatics Institute, Keck School of Medicine of USC, University of Southern California, Siemens Healthcare, Los Angeles, California, USA

ALLISON M. MCKENDRICK, PhD
Professor, C/O Department of Optometry and Vision Sciences, Department of Optometry and Vision Sciences, The University of Melbourne, Parkville, Victoria, Australia

RAJIV G. MENON, PhD
Research Scientist, Department of Radiology, NYU Langone Health, Bernard and Irene Schwartz Center for Biomedical Imaging, New York, New York, USA

GREGORY J. METZGER, PhD
Center for Magnetic Resonance Research
(CMRR), University of Minnesota, Minneapolis,
Minnesota, USA

BRADFORD A. MOFFAT, PhD
Associate Professor, The Melbourne Brain
Centre Imaging Unit, Department of Radiology,
The University of Melbourne, Parkville, Victoria,
Australia

MELANIE A. MORRISON, PhD
Department of Radiology and Biomedical
Imaging, University of California, San
Francisco, San Francisco, California, USA

BAO N. NGUYEN, PhD
Lecturer, C/O Department of Optometry and
Vision Sciences, Department of Optometry and
Vision Sciences, The University of Melbourne,
Parkville, Victoria, Australia

ROGER J. ORDIDGE, PhD
Professor, The Melbourne Brain Centre
Imaging Unit, Department of Radiology, The
University of Melbourne, Parkville, Victoria,
Australia

DANIEL PAECH, MD, MS
Division of Radiology, German Cancer
Research Center (DKFZ), Heidelberg, Germany

ALEXANDER RADBRUCH, MD, JD
Clinic for Diagnostic and Interventional
Neuroradiology, Bonn, Germany

RAVINDER R. REGATTE, PhD
Professor, Department of Radiology, NYU
Langone Health, Bernard and Irene Schwartz
Center for Biomedical Imaging, New York, New
York, USA

FARSHID SEPEHRBAND, PhD
Assistant Professor, Laboratory of Neuro
Imaging, Stevens Neuroimaging and
Informatics Institute, Keck School of Medicine
of USC, University of Southern California, Los
Angeles, California, USA

XINGFENG SHAO, PhD
Laboratory of FMRI Technology (LOFT), USC
Mark & Mary Stevens Neuroimaging and
Informatics Institute, Keck School of Medicine
of USC, University of Southern California, Los
Angeles, California, USA

ARTHUR W. TOGA, PhD
Director, Laboratory of Neuro Imaging,
Stevens Neuroimaging and Informatics
Institute, Keck School of Medicine of USC,
University of Southern California, Los Angeles,
California, USA

ELIZABETH TONG, MD
Assistant Professor, Department of Radiology,
Stanford, California, USA

KAMIL UǦURBIL, PhD
Center for Magnetic Resonance Research
(CMRR), University of Minnesota, Minneapolis,
Minnesota, USA

**PIERRE-FRANCOIS VAN DE MOORTELE,
MD, PhD**
Center for Magnetic Resonance Research
(CMRR), University of Minnesota, Minneapolis,
Minnesota, USA

GAURAV VERMA, PhD
Senior Scientist, Biomedical Engineering and
Imaging Institute, Icahn School of Medicine at
Mount Sinai, New York, New York, USA

DANNY J.J. WANG, PhD, MSCE
Laboratory of FMRI Technology (LOFT), USC
Mark & Mary Stevens Neuroimaging and
Informatics Institute, Department of Neurology,
Keck School of Medicine of USC, University of
Southern California, Los Angeles, California,
USA

KAI WANG, BS
Laboratory of FMRI Technology (LOFT), USC
Mark & Mary Stevens Neuroimaging and
Informatics Institute, Keck School of Medicine
of USC, University of Southern California, Los
Angeles, California, USA

LIRONG YAN, PhD
Laboratory of FMRI Technology (LOFT), USC
Mark & Mary Stevens Neuroimaging and
Informatics Institute, Department of Neurology,
Keck School of Medicine of USC, University of
Southern California, Los Angeles, California,
USA

VIVEK YEDAVALLI, MD, MS
Clinical Instructor, Department of Radiology,
Stanford University, Stanford, California, USA;
Assistant Professor of Radiology and
Radiological Sciences, Division of
Neuroradiology, Johns Hopkins University,
Baltimore, Maryland, USA

MICHAEL ZEINEH, MD, PhD
Associate Professor, Associate Chief of
Neuroradiology for Operations and IT,
Department of Radiology, Stanford University,
Lucas Center for Imaging, Stanford, California,
USA

Contents

Foreword   xiii

Suresh K. Mukherji

**Preface: Ultrahigh Field 7 T MR Imaging: Bridging the Gap Between Microscopic and
Systems Level Macroscopic Imaging**   xv

Meng Law

Neuroimaging at 3T vs 7T: Is It Really Worth It?   1

Stephen E. Jones, Jonathan Lee, and Meng Law

Food and Drug Administration approval of 7T MR imaging allows ultrahigh-field neu-roimaging to extend from the research realm into the clinical realm. Increased signal is clinically advantageous for smaller voxels and thereby high spatial resolution im-aging, with additional advantages of increased tissue contrast. Susceptibility, time-of-flight signal, and blood oxygen level–dependent signal also have favorable clinical benefit from 7T. This article provides a survey of clinical cases showcasing some ad-vantages of 7T.

**High-resolution Structural Magnetic Resonance Imaging and Quantitative Susceptibility
Mapping**   13

Vivek Yedavalli, Phillip DiGiacomo, Elizabeth Tong, and Michael Zeineh

High-resolution 7-T imaging and quantitative susceptibility mapping produce greater anatomic detail compared with conventional strengths because of improve-ments in signal/noise ratio and contrast. The exquisite anatomic details of deep structures, including delineation of microscopic architecture using advanced tech-niques such as quantitative susceptibility mapping, allows improved detection of abnormal findings thought to be imperceptible on clinical strengths. This article re-views caveats and techniques for translating sequences commonly used on 1.5 or 3 T to high-resolution 7-T imaging. It discusses for several broad disease categories how high-resolution 7-T imaging can advance the understanding of various dis-eases, improve diagnosis, and guide management.

UltraHigh Field MR Imaging in Epilepsy   41

Gaurav Verma, Bradley N. Delman, and Priti Balchandani

More than one million people in the United States suffer from seizures that are not controlled with antiseizure medications. Targeted interventions such as surgery and deep brain stimulation can confer seizure reduction or even freedom in many of these patients with drug-resistant epilepsy, but success critically depends on identification of epileptogenic zones through MR imaging. Ultrahigh field imaging fa-cilitates improved sensitivity and resolution across many imaging modalities and may facilitate better detection of epileptic markers than is achieved at lower field strengths. The increasing availability and clinical adoption of ultrahigh field scanners play an important role in characterizing drug-resistant epilepsy and planning for its treatment.

High-Resolution Neurovascular Imaging at 7T: Arterial Spin Labeling Perfusion, 4-Dimensional MR Angiography, and Black Blood MR Imaging   53

Xingfeng Shao, Lirong Yan, Samantha J. Ma, Kai Wang, and Danny J.J. Wang

Ultrahigh field offers increased resolution and contrast for neurovascular imaging. Arterial spin labeling methods benefit from an increased intrinsic signal-to-noise ratio of MR imaging signal and a prolonged tracer half-life at ultrahigh field, allowing the visualization of layer-dependent microvascular perfusion. Arterial spin labeling–based time-resolved 4-dimensional MR angiography at 7T provides a detailed depiction of the vascular architecture and dynamic blood flow pattern with high spatial and temporal resolutions. High-resolution black blood MR imaging at 7T allows detailed characterization of small perforating arteries such as lenticulostriate arteries. All techniques benefit from advances in parallel radiofrequency transmission technologies at ultrahigh field.

Perivascular Space Imaging at Ultrahigh Field MR Imaging   67

Giuseppe Barisano, Meng Law, Rachel M. Custer, Arthur W. Toga, and Farshid Sepehrband

The recent Food and Drug Administration approval of 7 T MR imaging scanners for clinical use has introduced the possibility to study the brain not only in physiologic but also in pathologic conditions at ultrahigh field (UHF). Because UHF MR imaging offers higher signal-to-noise ratio and spatial resolution compared with lower field clinical scanners, the benefits of UHF MR imaging are particularly evident for imaging small anatomic structures, such as the cerebral perivascular spaces (PVS). In this article, the authors describe the application of UHF MR imaging for the investigation of PVS.

Dynamic Glucose-Enhanced MR Imaging   77

Daniel Paech and Alexander Radbruch

Conventional medical imaging techniques use contrast agents that are chemically labeled, for example, iodine in the case of computed tomography, radioisotopes in the case of PET, or gadolinium in the case of MR imaging to create or enhance signal contrast and to visualize tissue compartments and features. Dynamic glucose-enhanced MR imaging represents a novel technique that uses natural, unlabeled d-glucose as a nontoxic biodegradable contrast agent in chemical exchange–sensitive MR imaging approaches.

7-T Magnetic Resonance Imaging in the Management of Brain Tumors   83

Melanie A. Morrison and Janine M. Lupo

This article provides an overview of the current status of ultrahigh-field 7-T magnetic resonance (MR) imaging in neuro-oncology, specifically for the management of patients with brain tumors. It includes a discussion of areas across the pretherapeutic, peritherapeutic, and posttherapeutic stages of patient care where 7-T MR imaging is currently being exploited and holds promise. This discussion includes existing technical challenges, barriers to clinical integration, as well as our impression of the future role of 7-T MR imaging as a clinical tool in neuro-oncology.

MR-EYE: High-Resolution MRI of the Human Eye and Orbit at Ultrahigh Field (7T)   103

 Video content accompanies this article at http://www.mri.theclinics.com.

Rebecca K. Glarin, Bao N. Nguyen, Jon O. Cleary, Scott C. Kolbe, Roger J. Ordidge, Bang V. Bui, Allison M. McKendrick, and Bradford A. Moffat

Ultrahigh-field (7T) MRI provides improved contrast and a signal-to-noise gain compared with lower magnetic field strengths. Here, we demonstrate feasibility and optimization of anatomic imaging of the eye and orbit using a dedicated commercial multichannel transmit and receive eye coil. Optimization of participant setup techniques and MRI sequence parameters allowed for improvements in the image resolution and contrast, and the eye and orbit coverage with minimal susceptibility and motion artifacts in a clinically feasible protocol.

Musculoskeletal MR Imaging Applications at Ultra-High (7T) Field Strength   117

Rajiv G. Menon, Gregory Chang, and Ravinder R. Regatte

Regulatory approval of ultrahigh field (UHF) MR imaging scanners for clinical use has opened new opportunities for musculoskeletal imaging applications. UHF MR imaging has unique advantages in terms of signal-to-noise ratio, contrast-to-noise ratio, spectral resolution, and multinuclear applications, thus providing unique information not available at lower field strengths. But UHF also comes with a set of technical challenges that are yet to be resolved and may not be suitable for all imaging applications. This review focuses on the latest research in musculoskeletal MR imaging applications at UHF including morphologic imaging, T_2, T_2^*, and $T_{1\rho}$ mapping, chemical exchange saturation transfer, sodium imaging, and phosphorus spectroscopy imaging applications.

Progress in Imaging the Human Torso at the Ultrahigh Fields of 7 and 10.5 T   e1

Kamil Uğurbil, Pierre-Francois Van de Moortele, Andrea Grant, Edward J. Auerbach, Arcan Ertürk, Russell Lagore, Jutta M. Ellermann, Xiaoxuan He, Gregor Adriany, and Gregory J. Metzger

Especially after the launch of 7 T, the ultrahigh magnetic field (UHF) imaging community achieved critically important strides in our understanding of the physics of radiofrequency interactions in the human body, which in turn has led to solutions for the challenges posed by such UHFs. As a result, the originally obtained poor image quality has progressed to the high-quality and high-resolution images obtained at 7 T and now at 10.5 T in the human torso. Despite these tremendous advances, work still remains to further improve the image quality and fully capitalize on the potential advantages UHF has to offer.

MAGNETIC RESONANCE IMAGING CLINICS OF NORTH AMERICA

FORTHCOMING ISSUES

May 2021
Advances in Diffusion-weighted Imaging
Kei Yamada, *Editor*

August 2021
MR Imaging of Chronic Liver Diseases and Liver Cancer
Khaled M. Elsayes and Claude B. Sirlin, *Editors*

November 2021
Pediatric Neuroimaging: State-of-the-Art
Mai-Lan Ho, *Editor*

RECENT ISSUES

November 2020
MR Safety
Robert E. Watson, *Editor*

August 2020
Advanced MR Techniques for Imaging the Abdomen and Pelvis
Sudhakar K. Venkatesh, *Editor*

May 2020
MR Imaging of the Shoulder
Naveen Subhas and Soterios Gyftopoulos, *Editors*

VISIT THE CLINICS ONLINE!
Access your subscription at:
www.theclinics.com

PROGRAM OBJECTIVE

The goal of *Magnetic Resonance Imaging Clinics of North America* is to keep practicing physicians up to date with current clinical practice by providing timely articles reviewing the state of the art in patient care.

TARGET AUDIENCE

All practicing physicians and healthcare professionals who provide patient care utilizing findings from Magnetic Resonance Imaging.

LEARNING OBJECTIVES

Upon completion of this activity, participants will be able to:

1. Review advances in ultra-high field (UHF) 7T neuroimaging in comparison to previous technology.
2. Discuss feasibility and optimisation of anatomical imaging of the eye and orbit using a dedicated commercial multichannel transmit and receive eye coil.
3. Recognize existing technical challenges, barriers to clinical integration, and the future role of 7T MRI as a clinical tool in neuro-oncology.

ACCREDITATION

The Elsevier Office of Continuing Medical Education (EOCME) is accredited by the Accreditation Council for Continuing Medical Education (ACCME) to provide continuing medical education for physicians.

The EOCME designates this journal-based CME activity enduring material for a maximum of 10 *AMA PRA Category 1 Credit*(s)™. Physicians should claim only the credit commensurate with the extent of their participation in the activity.

All other healthcare professionals requesting continuing education credit for this enduring material will be issued a certificate of participation.

DISCLOSURE OF CONFLICTS OF INTEREST

The EOCME assesses conflict of interest with its instructors, faculty, planners, and other individuals who are in a position to control the content of CME activities. All relevant conflicts of interest that are identified are thoroughly vetted by EOCME for fair balance, scientific objectivity, and patient care recommendations. EOCME is committed to providing its learners with CME activities that promote improvements or quality in healthcare and not a specific proprietary business or a commercial interest.

The planning committee, staff, authors and editors listed below have identified no financial relationships or relationships to products or devices they or their spouse/life partner have with commercial interest related to the content of this CME activity:

Gregor Adriany, PhD; Edward J. Auerbach, PhD; Giuseppe Barisano, MD; Bang V. Bui, PhD; Gregory Chang, MD; Regina Chavous-Gibson, MSN, RN; Jon O. Cleary, MD, PhD; Rachel M. Custer, MS; Bradley N. Delman, MD, MS; Phillip DiGiacomo, MS; Jutta M. Ellermann, MD, PhD; Rebecca K. Glarin, PGDipMRI; Andrea Grant, ScD; Xiaoxuan He, ME; Scott C. Kolbe, PhD; Pradeep Kuttysankaran; Russell Lagore, PhD; Meng Law, MBBS, FRANZCR, MD, FASFNR; Jonathan Lee, MD; Samantha J. Ma, PhD; Rajiv G. Menon, PhD; Gregory J. Metzger, PhD; Bradford A. Moffat, PhD; Melanie A. Morrison, PhD; Suresh K. Mukherji, MD, MBA, FACR; Bao N. Nguyen, PhD; Roger J. Ordidge, PhD; Daniel Paech, MD, MS; Alexander Radbruch, MD, JD; Ravinder R. Regatte, PhD; Farshid Sepehrband, PhD; Xingfeng Shao, PhD; Lynne S. Steinbach, MD, FACR; Arthur W. Toga, PhD; Elizabeth Tong, MD; Kamil Uğurbil, PhD; Pierre-Francois Van de Moortele, MD, PhD; John Vassallo; Gaurav Verma, PhD; Danny J.J. Wang, PhD, MSCE; Kai Wang, BS; Lirong Yan, PhD; Vivek Yedavalli, MD, MS.

The planning committee, staff, authors and editors listed below have identified financial relationships or relationships to products or devices they or their spouse/life partner have with commercial interest related to the content of this CME activity:

Priti Balchandani, PhD: holds patents/receives royalties from General Electric Company, Koninklijke Philips N.V., and Siemens

Arcan Ertürk, PhD: is employed by Medtronic

Stephen E. Jones, MD, PhD: receives research support from Biogen and is a consultant/advisor for Eisai Co., Ltd and Monteris

Janine M. Lupo, PhD: receives research support from General Electric Company

Allison M. McKendrick, PhD: receives research support from Heidelberg Engineering GmBH

Michael Zeineh, MD, PhD: receives research support from General Electric Company

UNAPPROVED/OFF-LABEL USE DISCLOSURE

The EOCME requires CME faculty to disclose to the participants:

1. When products or procedures being discussed are off-label, unlabelled, experimental, and/or investigational (not US Food and Drug Administration [FDA] approved); and
2. Any limitations on the information presented, such as data that are preliminary or that represent ongoing research, interim analyses, and/or unsupported opinions. Faculty may discuss information about pharmaceutical agents that is outside of FDA-approved labelling. This information is intended solely for CME and is not intended to promote off-label use of these

medications. If you have any questions, contact the medical affairs department of the manufacturer for the most recent prescribing information.

TO ENROLL
To enroll in the *Magnetic Resonance Imaging Clinics of North America* Continuing Medical Education program, call customer service at 1-800-654-2452 or sign up online at http://www.theclinics.com/home/cme. The CME program is available to subscribers for an additional annual fee of USD 281.00.

METHOD OF PARTICIPATION
In order to claim credit, participants must complete the following:
1. Complete enrolment as indicated above.
2. Read the activity.
3. Complete the CME Test and Evaluation. Participants must achieve a score of 70% on the test. All CME Tests and Evaluations must be completed online.

CME INQUIRIES/SPECIAL NEEDS
For all CME inquiries or special needs, please contact elsevierCME@elsevier.com.

Foreword

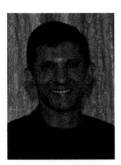

Suresh K. Mukherji, MD, MBA, FACR
Consulting Editor

Dr Meng Law beautifully framed this issue as "7.0 T versus 3.0 T." The only addition I would make is "7.0 T versus 1.5 T," since the majority of magnets in use globally are 1.5 T. There has been a gradual transition to 3.0 T, but not as rapidly as once predicted due to a myriad of reasons. The question is whether 7.0 T is ready for "prime time."

This issue of *Magnetic Resonance Imaging Clinics of North America* makes a compelling case for the future role of 7.0 T in a variety of clinical applications, including evaluation of brain tumors, epilepsy, multiple sclerosis, and orbital and musculoskeletal imaging. There are also several articles focusing on advantages of 7 T for various techniques, including functional MR imaging, susceptibility, and vascular imaging. The articles are superb; the author list is a "Who's Who" in their domain expertise, and the image quality is spectacular.

Finally, I would like to thank Dr Meng Law for editing this important issue. Meng and I have been colleagues and friends for many years, and it has been wonderful watching his career grow over the past 20 years. We have shared numerous "spirits" and rounds of golf on many occasions. Meng, I would like to take you up on your offer in the Preface and invite you to guest edit an issue of *Magnetic Resonance Imaging Clinics of North America* entitled "12.0 T versus 7.0 T" … due in 2035!

Suresh K. Mukherji, MD, MBA, FACR
Clinical Professor, Marian University
Director of Head & Neck Radiology
ProScan Imaging
Regional Medical Director
Envision Physician Services
Carmel, Indiana, USA

E-mail address:
sureshmukherji@hotmail.com

Magn Reson Imaging Clin N Am 29 (2021) xiii
https://doi.org/10.1016/j.mric.2020.09.011
1064-9689/21/© 2020 Published by Elsevier Inc.

Preface

Ultrahigh Field 7 T MR Imaging: Bridging the Gap Between Microscopic and Systems Level Macroscopic Imaging

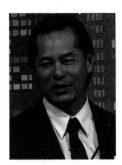

Meng Law, MBBS, FRANZCR, MD, FASFNR
Editor

Fourteen years ago, *Neuroimaging Clinics* published an issue entitled "3.0 T versus 1.5 T Imaging." This current issue represents a sequel that could be entitled "7.0 T versus 3.0 T Imaging." In year 2035, we may see an issue entitled "12.0 T versus 7.0 T Imaging" or perhaps more likely "AI-Powered Hybrid 12.0 T MR Imaging–CT-PET Scanner and Theranostic Focused US-Radio-Laser" all in one.

In the first article, we ask the question of whether 7 T is really worth it? I think putting together this issue of *Magnetic Resonance Imaging Clinics of North America* was well and truly worth it, particularly as 2020 has been an extremely challenging year for all of us, including my colleagues and friends who stoically contributed. I am extremely proud of this issue of *Magnetic Resonance Imaging Clinics of North America*, as it really does feature the absolute state-of-the-art ultra high field (UHF) 7 T MR imaging from leaders in our field. I believe we are now at the cusp of bridging super-high-resolution in vivo macroscopic MR imaging to systems level mesoscale imaging, to microscopic and physiologic imaging. This along with the installation of clinical MR imaging systems globally will now allow the translation of this technology into the clinic for imaging microscale pathology. The higher microscopic resolution demonstrates anatomy and pathology

that is not only previously invisible to the human eye but only detectable at a pixel level with machine learning algorithms. Deep learning and neural network approaches will make precision diagnoses possible with application of artificial or augmented intelligence analyses of combined hybrid multimodal imaging systems, pathologic, genomics, biofluid, and clinical digital health data science for individual patients. I sincerely hope we will see the beginnings of this in our lifetime and extend life expectancy beyond our dreams by the end of this century. Artificial or augmented intelligence will change not only health care but also every aspect of human existence.

Highlights in this issue include the UHF MR of the human eye and orbit, which provides an example of combining coil technology with very simple reproducible participant preparation techniques to reduce motion of the eye by taping the imaged eye shut and allowing the contralateral eye to fixate on the mirror and fixation target LCD screens. I believe we are presenting the highest-resolution in vivo human MR eye images published to date. UHF MR also demonstrates its advantage with superior visualization and quantitation of perivascular spaces and small lenticulostriate vessels, which we could barely "see" 20 years ago at 1.5 T but now routinely seen at 3 T. This issue also highlights extremely comprehensive

Magn Reson Imaging Clin N Am 29 (2021) xv–xvi
https://doi.org/10.1016/j.mric.2020.09.010
1064-9689/21/© 2020 Published by Elsevier Inc.

UHF imaging of brain tumors, epilepsy, musculo-skeletal as well as some of the most exquisite high-resolution UHF MR imaging of anatomic structures and myelin exploiting the advantages of susceptibility imaging at 7 T. The ability to visualize the subthalamic nuclei and other structures at 7 T allows direct targeting with deep brain stimulation and other novel therapeutic approaches again advancing the field of theranostics.

Finally, I would like to dedicate this issue of *Magnetic Resonance Imaging Clinics of North America* to all my friends and colleagues who have endured this year, particularly those who have contributed, my parents Sue and Lawrence, as well as Sol, who has been a beacon of light during these challenging times.

Meng Law, MBBS, FRANZCR, MD, FASFNR
Department of Radiology
Alfred Health
55 Commercial Road
Melbourne, Victoria 3004, Australia

E-mail address:
meng.law@monash.edu

Neuroimaging at 3T vs 7T
Is It Really Worth It?

Stephen E. Jones, MD, PhD[a],*, Jonathan Lee, MD[a], Meng Law, MD[b,c,d]

KEYWORDS

• Ultrahigh-field (UHF) MR imaging • 7T • Brain • Neuroimaging

KEY POINTS

• MR imaging at 7T provides greater signal-to-noise ratio, smaller voxel size, and/or faster scan times compared with 1.5T and 3T scans, at the expense of increased cost and artifact in certain applications.
• The primary clinical benefit of 7T MR imaging is problem solving when the resolution or signal of lower field strength magnets is not sufficient (eg, identifying subtle cortical dysplasia or the central vein sign in multiple sclerosis).
• Improvements in artifact reduction and the introduction of additional coils could make 7T more widely adopted in clinical settings.

INTRODUCTION

Over the past 30 years, clinical MR imaging has been demonstrated to be an essential component of medicine, and, with continuing research and development, the capabilities of this modality are still expanding. Increasing field strength is one of the improvements that has been made to this technology, as evidenced by the Food and Drug Administration (FDA) approval of a clinical 7T MR imaging system in 2017. Although 7T MR images have been available well before 2017 for research purposes, this approval now extends 7T imaging into the clinical realm.[1,2] This advance follows previous increases in field strength, with 1.5T systems approved in 1986 and 3T systems approved in 1998.[3] The 19-year interval between the approvals of 3T and 7T systems suggests that the next large increase in clinical field strength is much further in the future, and only recently have research MR imaging systems obtained field strengths higher than 7T for research (including a 10.5T system at the University of Minnesota,[4] an 11.7T system at the NeuroSpin Center at CEA Saclay, and an 11.7T

magnet at the National Institutes of Health). Therefore, the FDA-approved 7T technology currently available may represent the status of ultrahigh-field clinical imaging for some time to come.

This increased field strength necessarily comes with increased costs, however, including costs associated with more stringent siting requirements and coil expenses. These additional costs will mean that fewer units are sold, decreasing the discount that might come with scalability. Although 7T images may be exquisite compared with 3T images, this nonnegligible added capital expense for 7T mandates an assessment regarding the utility of 7T in a clinical setting. In the research setting, there are undoubted benefits to using 7T, but in the clinical world, is it really worth it?

Fig. 1 shows an approximate barometer of human academic research using 7T over the previous 9 years, using PubMed searches for the term, "7T." This graph shows a near-linear increase in the number of publications per year. If the term "clinical" is added, this number is reduced to approximately 25% of the total, but this fraction has been

[a] Section of Neuroradiology, Imaging Institute, Cleveland Clinic, 9500 Euclid Avenue, Cleveland, OH 44118, USA; [b] Department of Radiology, Alfred Health, The Alfred Centre, Level 1, 99 Commercial Road, Melbourne, Victoria 3004, Australia; [c] Department of Neuroscience, Monash University, Melbourne, Victoria, Australia; [d] Department of Electrical and Computer Systems Engineering, Monash University, Melbourne, Victoria, Australia
* Corresponding author.
E-mail address: joness19@ccf.org

Magn Reson Imaging Clin N Am 29 (2021) 1–12
https://doi.org/10.1016/j.mric.2020.09.001

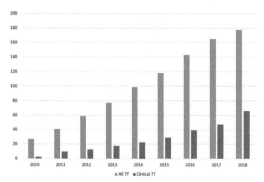

Fig. 1. Increase of annual publications mentioning the use of 7T in both the research realm (*blue bars*) and the clinical realm (*orange bars*). (*Data from* PubMed. Search results for the terms "7T" only versus "7T" and "clinical." Available at: https://pubmed.ncbi. nlm.nih.gov/.)

increasing in recent years, suggesting that 7T increasingly is used in the clinical realm.

Because the introduction of clinical 7T is too recent for a body of literature to have been established regarding cost effectiveness and return on investment, this article qualitatively explores the benefits of clinical 7T imaging by presenting a collection of clinical vignettes showing how 7T clinical imaging affected a patient's care. The advantages of 7T must be balanced, however, against its drawbacks, as discussed later.

Fourteen years ago, *Neuroimaging Clinics* published an issue entitled "3.0T versus 1.5T Imaging."[5] This current edition represents a sequel that could be entitled, "7.0T versus 3.0T Imaging." Subsequent articles cover various advanced imaging techniques using 7T. These techniques include quantitative susceptibility mapping at 7T, which has the potential to quantify the amount of intracranial amyloid-β aggregates in Alzheimer disease[6]; arterial spin labeling and dynamic contrast-enhanced perfusion techniques, which would benefit from contrast-to-noise ratio (CNR) improvements at 7T[7,8]; and 7T sodium imaging, which can be used to evaluate subtle cartilage loss[9] or early radiotherapy-induced cellular necrosis.[10] Additionally, 7T applications are discussed in detail, including 7T imaging of the human eye; imaging of nonlesional epilepsy, multiple sclerosis (MS), and brain tumors; vascular, perfusion, and permeability imaging; glutamate-weighted imaging; musculoskeletal and body applications; and simultaneous MR imaging with PET.

ADVANTAGES OF 7T IMAGING
Smaller Voxels

One of the principal advantages of increased magnetic field strength stems from the corresponding near-linear increase of signal-to-noise ratio (SNR).[11,12] This increased signal can be spent in several ways: obtaining smoother images by keeping the voxel the same volume, acquiring higher-resolution images with the same SNR because of the smaller voxels, and achieving faster scan times by keeping the voxels the same volume but reducing the number of averages, resulting in the same SNR. In practice, these 3 factors can be traded off against each other. **Fig. 2** shows 3T and 7T fluid-attenuated inversion recovery (FLAIR) images obtained from the same patient using the same voxel sizes. As expected, the 7T image is much smoother because of the increased SNR. For diagnostic purposes, this increased smoothness may not add much clinical information, and therefore the increased signal might be better used to obtain smaller voxels while maintaining the SNR of the 3T image.

Along with higher in-plane resolution, smaller voxels provide thinner sections. **Fig. 3** shows images from 1.5T gradient-recalled echo (GRE) and 7T susceptibility-weighted imaging (SWI) scans from a patient evaluated for traumatic brain injury (TBI) with several known chronic microhemorrhages in the left frontal lobe. The same span of 5 1.5T images is covered by 32 7T images. This enables visualization of the microhemorrhages, previously thought to be multiple and separate, as being linearly connected, representing either a developmental venous anomaly or hemorrhage into a perivascular space. Although the compared images are not exactly the same (GRE vs SWI), **Fig. 3** illustrates one of the major benefits of clinical 7T imaging: better visualization of smaller structures.[13–16]

Increased Contrast-to-Noise Ratio

Tissue relaxation times also favorably scale with field strength, leading to increased CNR.[12] Additional improvement is seen from less partial volume averaging. Altogether, 7T can increase the conspicuity between different brain regions or between a lesion and normal brain. An example of the former is shown in **Fig. 4**, which shows 3T and 7T T1-weighted volumetric images from the same patient in coregistered planes. At 7T, the ratio of gray matter to white matter signal is increased, improving the conspicuity of the gray-white junction. This could improve detection of focal cortical dysplasias in patients with epilepsy. Another CNR advantage of 7T is increased sensitivity to susceptibility changes. As shown in **Fig. 3**, 7T offers the benefit not only of smaller voxels but also of increased conspicuity of signal dephasing from susceptibility effects from hemosiderin. This

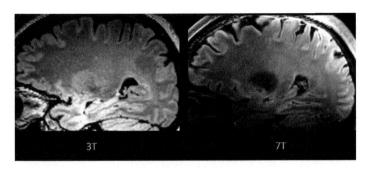

Fig. 2. Comparison of sagittal FLAIR images from the same patient. Images were obtained at 3T (left) and 7T (right) field strengths, using the same sequence with the same slice thickness and inplane voxel size. The 7T image displays a smoother texture because of the increased SNR, with all other factors being the same.

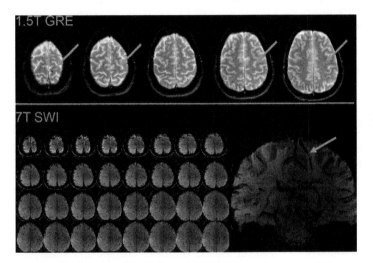

Fig. 3. Benefit of thinner axial sections. The images in the top panel are from a 44-year-old woman with postconcussive symptoms after falling off a horse 2 months earlier. These images were obtained on a clinical 1.5T MR imaging system, using a slice thickness of 4 mm. The images in the bottom left panel are from the same patient but were obtained at 7T, with 32 images spanning the same range as the 5 images in the top panel. The thinner sections allow for a reliable multiplanar reconstruction to demonstrate the linear relationship of the susceptibility foci (bottom right image).

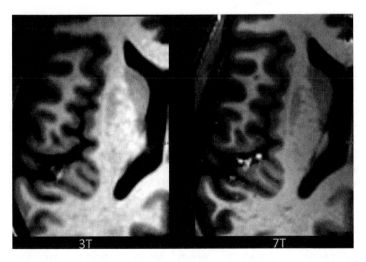

Fig. 4. Comparison of sagittal T1-weighted images with similar voxel size, using an MPRAGE for 3T (left) and MR2RAGE for 7T (right). Note the increased contrast ratio of gray matter to white matter at 7T, which increases the conspicuity of the grey-white junction.

increased sensitivity can enable improved detection of microhemorrhages,[13] which could be useful for diseases as TBI, amyloid angiopathy, and cavernous malformations.

Imaging for some diseases benefits from both smaller voxels and increased CNR. For example, MS lesions have heightened conspicuity on a 7T magnetization prepared – rapid gradient echo, with two readouts (MP2RAGE) image, and smaller voxels can enable evaluation of the integrity of the subcortical U-fibers. A synergistic benefit from susceptibility effects is the ability to identify the central vein in MS lesions. Epilepsy evaluation also can benefit from both smaller voxels and increased CNR, with increased conspicuity of small cortical-subcortical lesions.[17] Such identification can greatly affect patient care, allowing for faster identification of surgical targets for resection, more efficient placement of stereoelectroencephalography (SEEG) electrodes during an invasive evaluation, or the information needed to skip an invasive evaluation and proceed directly to resection.

Other Advantages

Imaging at 7T also offers benefits to sequences, such as MR angiography. For instance, high-resolution arterial time-of-flight (TOF) MR angiography at 7T allows better visualization of smaller intracranial arteries and cerebrovascular lesions, including small aneurysms[15]; 7T MR angiography has been shown to provide image quality at least equal to that obtained with digital subtraction angiography for imaging aneurysms[18] and arteriovenous malformations,[19] and 7T offers improvements over 3T for functional MR imaging, mostly by providing increased functional CNR with less partial volume effects and more distinct spatial features, allowing for descriptions of fine-scaled patterns[20] and better visualization of smaller neural circuits such as the ventral tegmental area in patients with major depressive disorder.[21]

VIGNETTES DEMONSTRATING UTILITY OF CLINICAL 7T NEUROIMAGING
Example 1. Epilepsy (Focal Cortical Dysplasia)

The patient is an 18-year-old man who began having seizures at 6 years of age, with electroencephalogram (EEG) suggesting a left central origin. An fluorodeoxyglucose-PET study showed subtle mild hypometabolism in the left frontoparietal region, and an ictal single-photon emission computed tomography (CT) study showed possible sites of seizure within this general region; however, all of the previous 3T MR imaging scans

the patient had undergone had been unremarkable. Without a definitive target, an invasive evaluation was deferred and the patient was treated with medication. The patient's seizure frequency increased, however. Magnetoencephalography demonstrated spikes in the left frontal parietal operculum, but 3T MR imaging again showed no abnormality. A 7T MR imaging study showed blurring of the gray-white junction with abnormal T1 hypointensity in the subcortical white matter of the left frontal parietal operculum, consistent with cortical dysplasia (Fig. 5). With a definitive target identified, SEEG evaluation confirmed an epileptogenic focus at that location. Biopsy demonstrated a focal cortical dysplasia, and subsequent laser ablation greatly decreased the patient's seizure frequency.

Example 2. MR Angiography and Origin of Carotid Cave Aneurysm

The patient is a 51-year-old woman presenting with headache and bilateral facial and ear pain. Because the patient had a family history of aneurysm, 3T TOF MR angiography was performed. This examination demonstrated a small inferiorly and medially oriented internal carotid artery aneurysm in the carotid cave. Treatment of carotid cave aneurysms is controversial, because the location may be entirely extradural or may have an intradural component.[22] The patient was referred to a neurointerventionalist for a catheter angiogram; the physician opted to first perform high-resolution MR angiography using a 7T system (Fig. 6). Based on these images, the aneurysm takeoff was believed to be proximal to the ophthalmic artery and likely completely extradural. An immediate angiogram was deferred, and the patient is being followed clinically and with imaging.

Example 3. Large Vessel Vasculitis

The patient is a 50-year-old man with hypertension, hyperlipidemia, and diabetes who presented with acute infarcts that initially were thought to be embolic. No central cardiac or carotid etiology was found, and new small infarcts were seen in the right middle cerebral artery territory. Routine brain MR angiography showed multiple intracranial vessel irregularities, including in the right M1 segment; this finding was confirmed on conventional angiogram. A 3T vessel wall imaging protocol showed multiple areas of wall enhancement, including the right M1; however, it was unclear whether the wall enhancement was circumferential, which would indicate atherosclerosis, or eccentric, which would indicate vasculitis.

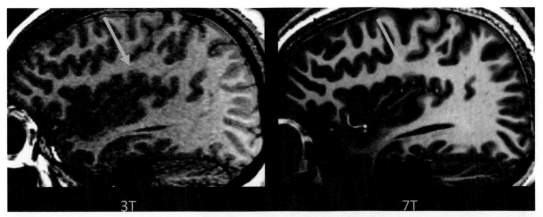

Fig. 5. Comparison of sagittal T1-weighted images using an MPRAGE for 3T (left) and MR2RAGE for 7T (right) shows increased conspicuity of the focal cortical dysplasia in the left frontal parietal operculum on 7T.

Therefore, 7T vessel wall imaging was performed. The smaller voxel size with 7T allowed for the confirmation of eccentric wall enhancement consistent with vasculitis (**Fig. 7**). The patient first was treated with methylprednisolone and then with cyclophosphamide, and subsequent biopsy of the subarachnoid vessels confirmed the diagnosis of primary angiitis of the central nervous system.

Example 4. Possible Cestode Infection

The patient is a 69-year-old woman with a history of lymphoma that had resolved with chemotherapy. She presented with recurrent fevers and altered mental status; 3T MR imaging of the brain showed multiple small peripheral enhancing lesions, not otherwise well defined. CT of the chest, abdomen, and pelvis also showed innumerable pulmonary nodules and spleen, liver, and renal

lesions. A parasitic disease was suspected, and 7T MR imaging was performed. The higher spatial resolution of this modality exquisitely demonstrated the eccentric T2 hypointense wall of a scolex (**Fig. 8**), which was suggestive of neurocysticercosis. The patient underwent an open liver biopsy and was treated with antiparasitic medication, after which she demonstrated clinical improvement. Subsequent DNA sequencing returned a result not of cysticercosis but of an infection caused by a closely related zoonotic cestode *Versteria* species.

Example 5. Multiple Sclerosis

The patient is a 21-year-old woman presenting with lower leg paresthesias that had progressed to her trunk and arms; 3T brain MR imaging showed multiple nonspecific white matter lesions, possibly compatible with MS. An MS neurologist

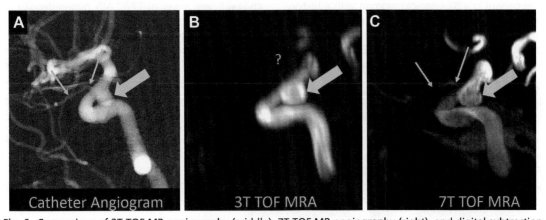

Fig. 6. Comparison of 3T TOF MR angiography (middle), 7T TOF MR angiography (right), and digital subtraction images from a catheter angiogram (left) of a carotid cave aneurysm (thick arrow). Note that improved spatial resolution on 7T TOF MR angiography, similar to the image from the catheter angiogram, shows the ophthalmic artery (small arrows), which is not visualized at 3T.

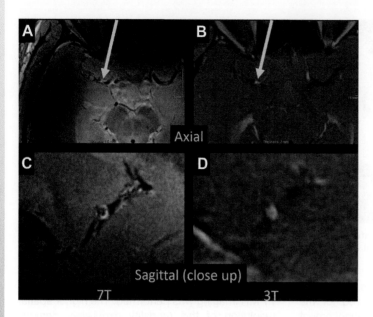

Fig. 7. Axial 3D (first row) and reconstructed sagittal (second row) fat and blood saturated T1 post contrast images were obtain at 3T and 7T. Note the eccentric wall enhancement in the right middle cerebral artery in this patient with vasculitis is much better appreciate on 7T images rather than 3T.

ordered 7T MR imaging using a T2* GRE sequence. The examination demonstrated a central vein extending through multiple lesions (**Fig. 9**), suggestive of MS. The patient was started on treatment with disease-modifying agents and is doing well. The lesions in this newly diagnosed patient were small with subtle features; in contrast, **Fig. 10** shows 3T and 7T images from a patient with advanced MS. In these images, the central veins coursing through most of the lesions are more obvious, particularly on 7T.

Example 6. Counterexample of White Matter Lesions: Central Nervous System Vasculopathy

The patient is a 52-year-old woman with a history of migraines, Sjögren disease, Behçet disease, and breast cancer who presented with migraines and lower extremity parasthesias. Brain MR imaging demonstrated multiple nonspecific white matter lesions in a pattern suggestive of MS. Subsequent 7T MR imaging also demonstrated these lesions, but relatively few of the lesions showed the central vein sign (**Fig. 11**). Based on these findings, the neurologist favored a diagnosis of Sjögren vasculopathy rather than MS.

Example 7. Progressive Multifocal Leukoencephalopathy

The patient is a 56-year-old man with a 32-year history of MS. After a long treatment course of interferon beta-1a caused increasing paresthesias, his medication was switched to natalizumab. During this treatment, the patient presented with worsening arm clumsiness, and brain MR imaging showed new areas of T2/FLAIR hyperintensity in the left frontal regions with a focus of enhancement. The pattern suggested progressive multifocal leukoencephalopathy (PML), with active demyelination less likely. An urgent lumbar

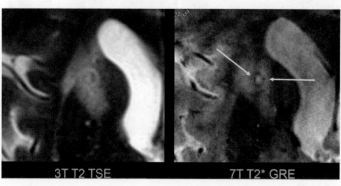

Fig. 8. Axial 3T T2 versus 7T T2* images showing better visualization of the T2 hypointense cyst wall (left arrow) and eccentric scolex (right arrow) from a cestode infection in the right basal ganglia on 7T.

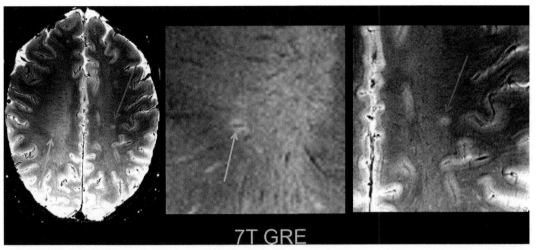

Fig. 9. Axial T2 GRE image on 7T showing multiple demyelinating plaques in a patient with MS (left panel). The middle and right panels are close-up images of two plaques shown by the arrows, demonstrating the central vein sign, which is specific for MS.

puncture was performed, however, and JC virus (JCV) was not detected by polymerase chain reaction, suggesting that this was not PML; 7T MR imaging showed a band of linear cortical susceptibility loss at the gray-white junction (**Fig. 12**), which had been noted before in other cases of PML imaged at 7T.[23] Based on this result, additional cerebrospinal fluid was sent to a dedicated PML laboratory, and 10 copies/mL of JCV DNA were identified. The patient was treated for natalizumab-related PML with urgent plasma exchange and is doing well.

Example 8. Improved Detection of Traumatic Brain Injury

The patient is a 55-year-old man who underwent head CT after a recent motor vehicle accident; the CT of the head did not reveal any abnormalities. Because the patient was experiencing worsening headaches, he presented to a TBI clinic, and brain MR imaging at 1.5T showed several small foci of susceptibility in the right frontal operculum region, possibly due to trauma, with other etiologies possible, such as hypertension or amyloid angiopathy. Because the patient continued to experience headaches, he was scanned at 7T. This study showed not only that the previous foci were linearly spread at the gray-white junction but also that additional foci were present in the left occipital lobe (**Fig. 13**). The neurologistconcluded, therefore, that the patient's symptoms were due to hemorrhagic axonal injury.

Note that the microbleeds in the left occipital lobe were retrospectively apparent on the 1.5T images, but they were only marginally conspicuous

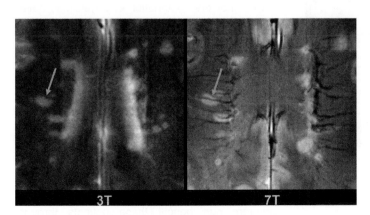

Fig. 10. Axial T2 images on 3T (left) versus 7T (right) T2 GRE showing multiple demyelinating plaques in a patient with MS, but the central vein sign is much better appreciated on 7T. One example plaque is indicated by the arrow.

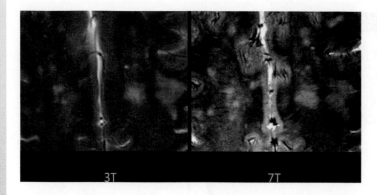

Fig. 11. Axial T2 images on 3T (left) versus 7T (right) T2 GRE showing multiple white matter changes in a patient with Sjögren syndrome. On the 7T images, there is better appreciation that very few lesions have the central vein sign, indicating that MS is unlikely.

at that field strength. This emphasizes that in addition to revealing de novo lesions not seen at lower field strengths, 7T also can increase the conspicuity of lesions that are present at lower field strengths but are insufficiently conspicuous for a neuroradiologist to reliably detect.

Example 9. Functional magnetic resonance imaging at 7T

The blood oxygen level–dependent (BOLD) signal is known to scale favorably with magnetic field strength, ranging between the linear and square of the field strength,[24] and many publications have described the advantages of using 7T for

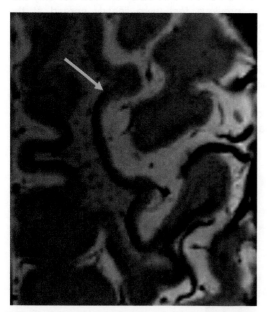

Fig. 12. Axial T2 GRE image on 7T showing linear cortical susceptibility at the gray-white matter junction (*white arrow*) of the left superior frontal gyrus, likely indicating PML as the cause of the T2 hyperintensity in the adjacent white matter.

BOLD functional MR imaging .[25–27] Just as higher signal strength from structural images can be used for different purposes, this increased BOLD signal also can be used in various ways. For example, in comparisons of BOLD functional MR imaging 3T and 7T images, the voxel size can be kept the same, with the increased BOLD signal used to enhance signal within these voxels; alternatively, the voxel size can be reduced to achieve a similar level of signal, albeit in smaller voxels. **Fig. 14** shows an example of these methods applied to a finger-tapping task. These images demonstrate robust activation in the hand knob; the activation is defined slightly better at 7T, but this increased definition does not add much to the evaluation (top row, middle column). The voxel size, however, can be reduced at 7T to show more clearly colocalization of BOLD activation with the cortical ribbon (top row, right column). For other brain structures with BOLD activation that typically is too weak to pass common statistical thresholds, the enhanced BOLD signal at 7T used with standard 3T voxel size can reveal otherwise weak foci. For instance, the thalamic nuclei associated with the finger-tapping task are not seen at 3T or 7T with small voxels but are seen clearly at 7T with larger voxels (bottom row). Research has shown that the contribution of physiologic noise to BOLD-weighted data also increases with field strength,[28] such that when using voxel sizes at 7T similar to those used at 3T, the noise dominates true BOLD signals. Thus, it generally is recommended to acquire BOLD-weighted data at a higher spatial resolution. Enhanced SNR from lower spatial resolution (eg, middle column) then can be achieved by spatially filtering the acquired data.

Clinical functional MR imaging has been approved by the FDA and generally is used for preoperative planning in patients with brain tumors and for evaluating eloquent cortex in patients with epilepsy. A clinical 7T functional MR imaging program can benefit these patients through

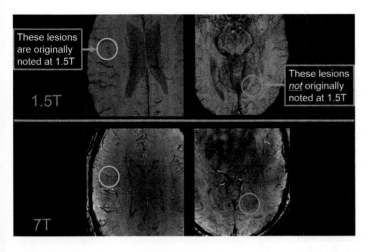

Fig. 13. Axial 1.5T SWI (top row) and 7T SWI (bottom row) images were obtained. Note that there is improved detection of multiple foci of susceptibility in a linear pattern in the right frontal operculum (left panels) and left occipital lobe (right panels) on 7T likely indicating hemorrhagic axonal injury due to trauma.

increased spatial localization or shorter scan times. Shorter scan times are advantageous especially in this population, because patients with tumors or epilepsy have a higher incidence of motion during scans, which can confound the analysis. With 7T, rather than using 4 blocks of finger tapping of language, only 2 or 3 blocks would be needed. Similarly, rather than 3 language paradigms, perhaps only 2 would be required.

DISADVANTAGES OF 7T

The greatest technical disadvantage of 7T is artifact caused by B0 and B1 inhomogeneity.[29] These artifacts can affect gradient-echo and spin-echo sequences differently, with B0 affecting gradient-echo images near air-tissue interfaces and B1 affecting spin-echo images more unpredictably. In addition, the radiofrequency penetration is less, with the shortened wavelength at 7T (13 cm) exciting spins more inhomogeneously. This contributes to a more complicated distribution of specific absorption rate, including hot spots, a factor that can affect safety as the specific absorption rate scales supralinearly with magnetic field.[25]

With 7T, there also is considerable signal loss in the inferior regions of the head, notably affecting the inferior and anterior regions of the temporal lobes, the sella, and orbits, all regions near osseous and air-filled structures. This can affect clinical imaging for conditions such as epilepsy,

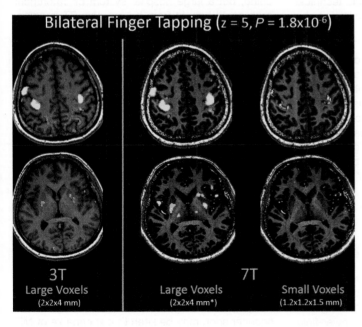

Fig. 14. Comparison of statistical maps from the same patient performing a bilateral finger-tapping functional MR imaging paradigm at 3T and 7T. The displayed images show two axial levels, through the hand knob (*top row*) and the thalamus (*bottom row*). With a threshold z-score of 5, images from the left column using 2 mm × 2 mm × 4 mm voxels at 3T show strong activation in the hand knob, with no activation in the thalamus. The middle column shows images with a corresponding voxel size of 2 mm × 2 mm × 4 mm at 7T, demonstrating strong activation in the hand knob and in the thalamus. With an acquired voxel size of 1.2 mm × 1.2 mm × 1.5 mm at 7T, images in the right column show strong activation in the hand knob that is clearly colocalized with the cortical ribbon. Thalamic activation, however, no longer is seen.

Alzheimer disease, and head and neck disease. Field distortions are greater at 7T than at 3T, which affects preoperative surgical planning requiring accurate stereotactic navigation. Although small voxels are a clear benefit for imaging lesions, their small size also makes them more susceptible to motion degradation.

The safety of scanning patients with implants at 7T is more uncertain than at lower field strengths, with concerns raised regarding dangerous torques, displacements, or local tissue heating.[30–32] In terms of research, a reluctance to scan healthy participants with implants is understandable, with the goal of avoiding any unnecessary risks. In a clinical practice, however, the risk-benefit balance shifts, requiring considering scanning patients with implants. Also, unlike the research population, the clinical patient population is far more likely to have implants. To this end, there now is a growing body of literature addressing the numerous classes of implants and the conditions under which they can be scanned.[33–42]

Among potential solutions for reducing B1 inhomogeneity effects is the incorporation of parallel transmit technologies, which permit more uniform B1 fields. Other improvements derive from higher order shimming capabilities and other advanced sequences to reduce flip angle nonuniformity over regions of interest.[25] A simpler method of reducing nonuniformity near-inferior regions of the head is the use of dielectric pads, but the improvement with this method is incomplete. The introduction of 3T MR imaging also was associated with its share of technical concerns,[43] which were addressed over time; many of the technical difficulties associated with 7T also are likely to be resolved eventually.

Increased siting requirements for 7T machines initially were a challenge because of concerns regarding unacceptable stray fields from the ultrahigh-field magnet; this problem was addressed passively through the use of large rooms with heavy wall shielding. Now with the availability of actively shielded magnets, the weight of the room and MR imaging system is much less, and the machine can be installed above the ground floor. Although the 7T MR imaging footprint is larger than that of a 3T, the system still can fit inside a room as small as 4.27 m × 9.14 m.

FUTURE DIRECTIONS FOR 7T NEUROIMAGING

At a cost of approximately $1 million per tesla, many clinical departments have to balance the acquisition of 1 7T MR imaging machine against the same funding supporting 3 to 6 lower-field

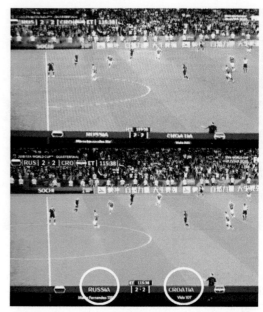

Fig. 15. Two views of the 2018 World Cup soccer game between Croatia and Russia. The top image is from a 2004 24-inches CRT television; the bottom image is from a modern 24-inches HDTV. Although the flow of the game can be appreciated on both displays, fine details, such as the team names and scores, can be appreciated only at high resolution.

MR imaging machines. As such, the clinical utility of 7T must be considered within a large fleet of lower-field clinical MR imaging systems. Perhaps not every hospital needs a 7T MR imaging machine, but a large hospital system or catchment area could benefit from having one; 7T imaging, therefore, may be used not as a first-line scanning modality but as a problem-solving tool.

There admittedly remain technical obstacles and room for improvement. Chief among these is field inhomogeneity, for which parallel transmission may offer useful solutions. Wang and colleagues demonstrate the benefits of parallel transmit coils in a clinical 7T MR imaging system. Other important unmet needs include the introduction of new 7T coils. The 7T system currently available is supplied with only a 32-channel receive/1-channel transmit brain coil and a 25-channel receive/1-channel transmit knee coil. For a neuroradiology practice, head and neck and spine coils are needed, and additional coils are needed for musculoskeletal, spine, and body applications. Technical difficulties must be overcome, however, before these coils are available.

Finally, considering recent advances in hybrid imaging technology and artificial intelligence, a scanner soon may be seen that is capable of MR imaging, PET, CT, ultrasound, and particle imaging and that will provide digital data that can be analyzed by artificial intelligence, providing superior diagnostic capabilities and perhaps even theranostics triage.

CONCLUSION

Neuroimaging at 7T is useful in the clinical setting but not necessarily for all patients and studies. The 3 main advantages of 7T over lower-field systems are higher spatial resolution, increased CNR for some sequences, and increased BOLD signal for functional studies. Therefore, 7T offers advantages for clinical cases requiring more detailed imaging of small pathologic features (eg, the presence of central vein sign in MS) or increased conspicuity of pathologic signal (eg, gray-white junction in focal cortical dysplasia) as well as for cases requiring functional MR imaging for preoperative planning. These advantages must be balanced, however, against the main drawbacks of 7T—cost, availability, and artifact.

Given the drawbacks of 7T imaging, this technique is best used not as a first-line imaging modality but as a problem-solving modality. That is, when more accessible lower-field imaging studies have been performed and questions remain, recourse to a 7T study is a reasonable option. Not all imaging requires the high level of detail offered by 7T, but a small fraction of studies will benefit and thereby alter a patient's clinical care. Sometimes details matter, and an analogy can be made with home television sets. For decades, televisions used cathode ray tubes (CRTs), which amply served the viewers' needs. Now CRT televisions have been replaced by high-definition televisions (HDTVs). **Fig. 15** compares similarly sized CRT and HDTV views showing the same scene from a World Cup soccer match. Although both television systems allow viewers to watch the flow of the game, sometimes details matter. For instance, the score and the names of the teams are difficult to discern on the CRT image but easy to read on the HDTV image. Similarly, 7T imaging could be viewed as high-definition MR imaging.

DISCLOSURE

SEJ: Biogen, Siemens, St Jude, Eisai, Monteris. JL: Nothing to disclose. ML: Nothing to disclose.

REFERENCES

1. van der Kolk AG, Hendrikse J, Zwanenburg JJ, et al. Clinical applications of 7 T MRI in the brain. Eur J Radiol 2013;82(5):708–18.

2. Balchandani P, Naidich TP. Ultra-high-field MR neuroimaging. AJNR Am J Neuroradiol 2015;36(7):1204–15.

3. Edelman RR. The history of MR imaging as seen through the pages of radiology. Radiology 2014;273(2S):S181–200.

4. He X, Ertürk MA, Grant A, et al. First in-vivo human imaging at 10.5 T: imaging the body at 447 MHz. Magn Reson Med 2020;84(1):289–303.

5. Roberts TPL. Preface. Neuroimaging Clin 2006;16(2):xv–xvi.

6. Tiepolt S, Schäfer A, Rullmann M, et al. Quantitative susceptibility mapping of amyloid-β aggregates in Alzheimer's disease with 7T MR. J Alzheimers Dis 2018;64(2):393–404.

7. Ivanov D, Gardumi A, Haast RA, et al. Comparison of 3 T and 7 T ASL techniques for concurrent functional perfusion and BOLD studies. Neuroimage 2017;156:363–76.

8. Menezes GL, Stehouwer BL, Klomp DW, et al. Dynamic contrast-enhanced breast MRI at 7T and 3T: an intra-individual comparison study. Springerplus 2016;5:13.

9. Maggiorelli F, Buonincontri G, Retico A, et al. Sodium imaging of the human knee cartilage with magnetic resonance at ultra high field: development of a double frequency (1 H/23 Na) RF coil. Paper presented at: 2017 International Applied Computational Electromagnetics Society Symposium-Italy (ACES), 2017.

10. Huang L, Zhang Z, Qu B, et al. Imaging of Sodium MRI for therapy evaluation of brain metastase with cyberknife at 7T: a case report. Cureus 2018;10(4):e2502.

11. Redpath TW. Signal-to-noise ratio in MRI. Br J Radiol 1998;71(847):704–7.

12. Duyn JH. The future of ultra-high field MRI and fMRI for study of the human brain. Neuroimage 2012;62(2):1241 8.

13. Obusez EC, Lowe M, Oh S-H, et al. 7T MR of intracranial pathology: preliminary observations and comparisons to 3T and 1.5 T. Neuroimage 2018;168:459–76.

14. De Ciantis A, Barba C, Tassi L, et al. 7T MRI in focal epilepsy with unrevealing conventional field strength imaging. Epilepsia 2016;57(3):445–54.

15. De Cocker LJ, Lindenholz A, Zwanenburg JJ, et al. Clinical vascular imaging in the brain at 7 T. Neuroimage 2018;168:452–8.

16. van Egmond SL, Visser F, Pameijer FA, et al. In vivo imaging of the inner ear at 7T MRI: image evaluation and comparison with 3T. Otol Neurotol 2015;36(4):687–93.

17. Feldman RE, Delman BN, Pawha PS, et al. 7T MRI in epilepsy patients with previously normal clinical MRI exams compared against healthy controls. PLoS One 2019;14(3):e0213642.

18. Matsushige T, Kraemer M, Schlamann M, et al. Ventricular microaneurysms in Moyamoya angiopathy visualized with 7T MR angiography. AJNR Am J Neuroradiol 2016;37(9):1669–72.

19. Wrede KH, Dammann P, Johst S, et al. Non-enhanced MR imaging of cerebral arteriovenous malformations at 7 Tesla. Eur Radiol 2016;26(3):829–39.

20. Vu AT, Jamison K, Glasser MF, et al. Tradeoffs in pushing the spatial resolution of fMRI for the 7T Human Connectome Project. Neuroimage 2017;154:23–32.

21. Morris LS, Kundu P, Costi S, et al. Ultra-high field MRI reveals mood-related circuit disturbances in depression: a comparison between 3-Tesla and 7-Tesla. Transl Psychiatry 2019;9(1):94.

22. Joo W, Funaki T, Yoshioka F, et al. Microsurgical anatomy of the carotid cave. Neurosurgery 2012;70(2 suppl operative):300–11.

23. Baldassari LE, Jones SE, Clifford DB, et al. Progressive multifocal leukoencephalopathy with extended natalizumab dosing. Neurol Clin Pract 2018;8(3):e12–4.

24. van der Zwaag W, Francis S, Head K, et al. fMRI at 1.5, 3 and 7 T: characterising BOLD signal changes. Neuroimage 2009;47(4):1425–34.

25. Uğurbil K. Magnetic resonance imaging at ultrahigh fields. IEEE Trans Biomed Eng 2014;61(5):1364–79.

26. Ladd ME, Bachert P, Meyerspeer M, et al. Pros and cons of ultra-high-field MRI/MRS for human application. Prog Nucl Magn Reson Spectrosc 2018;109:1–50.

27. Beisteiner R, Robinson S, Wurnig M, et al. Clinical fMRI: evidence for a 7T benefit over 3T. Neuroimage 2011;57(3):1015–21.

28. Triantafyllou C, Hoge RD, Krueger G, et al. Comparison of physiological noise at 1.5 T, 3 T and 7 T and optimization of fMRI acquisition parameters. Neuroimage 2005;26(1):243–50.

29. Truong T-K, Chakeres DW, Beversdorf DQ, et al. Effects of static and radiofrequency magnetic field inhomogeneity in ultra-high field magnetic resonance imaging. Magn Reson Imaging 2006;24(2):103–12.

30. Hoff MN, McKinney At, Shellock FG, et al. Safety considerations of 7-T MRI in clinical practice. Radiology 2019;292(3):509–18.

31. Kraff O, Quick HH. Safety of implants in high field and ultrahigh field MRI. Radiologe 2019;59(10):898–905.

32. Kraff O, Quick HH. 7T: physics, safety, and potential clinical applications. J Magn Reson Imaging 2017;46(6):1573–89.

33. Sammet CL, Yang X, Wassenaar PA, et al. RF-related heating assessment of extracranial neurosurgical implants at 7T. Magn Reson Imaging 2013;31(6):1029–34.

34. Dula AN, Virostko J, Shellock FG. Assessment of MRI issues at 7 T for 28 implants and other objects. AJR Am J Roentgenol 2014;202(2):401–5.

35. Wezel J, Kooij BJ, Webb AG. Assessing the MR compatibility of dental retainer wires at 7 Tesla. Magn Reson Med 2014;72(4):1191–8.

36. Noureddine Y, Bitz AK, Ladd ME, et al. Experience with magnetic resonance imaging of human subjects with passive implants and tattoos at 7 T: a retrospective study. Magma 2015;28(6):577–90.

37. Feng DX, McCauley JP, Morgan-Curtis FK, et al. Evaluation of 39 medical implants at 7.0 T. Br J Radiol 2015;88(1056):20150633.

38. Chen B, Schoemberg T, Kraff O, et al. Cranial fixation plates in cerebral magnetic resonance imaging: a 3 and 7 Tesla in vivo image quality study. Magma 2016;29(3):389–98.

39. Oriso K, Kobayashi T, Sasaki M, et al. Impact of the static and radiofrequency magnetic fields produced by a 7T MR imager on metallic dental materials. Magn Reson Med Sci 2016;15(1):26–33.

40. Tsukimura I, Murakami H, Sasaki M, et al. Assessment of magnetic field interactions and radiofrequency-radiation-induced heating of metallic spinal implants in 7 T field. J Orthop Res 2017;35(8):1831–7.

41. Barisano G, Culo B, Shellock FG, et al. 7-Tesla MRI of the brain in a research subject with bilateral, total knee replacement implants: case report and proposed safety guidelines. Magn Reson Imaging 2019;57:313–6.

42. Culo B, Valencerina S, Law M, et al. Assessment of metallic patient support devices and other items at 7-Tesla: findings applied to 46 additional devices. Magn Reson Imaging 2019;57:250–3.

43. Willinek WA, Kuhl CK. 3.0 T neuroimaging: technical considerations and clinical applications. Neuroimaging Clin N Am 2006;16(2):217–28, ix.

High-resolution Structural Magnetic Resonance Imaging and Quantitative Susceptibility Mapping

Vivek Yedavalli, MD, MS[a,b], Phillip DiGiacomo, MS[c], Elizabeth Tong, MD[d], Michael Zeineh, MD, PhD[e,*]

KEYWORDS

- High-resolution 7 T • Quantitative susceptibility mapping • Motion correction
- Neurodegenerative diseases • Neuropsychiatric diseases • Hippocampus • Midbrain

KEY POINTS

- High-resolution 7 T allows greater anatomic detail compared with conventional strengths (3 T and 1.5 T) because of improvements in signal/noise ratio and contrast, in particular with iron-sensitive sequences such as quantitative susceptibility mapping.
- Motion-compensated sequences are key to taking advantage of this increased resolution.
- The greater anatomic detail allows increased detection of disorder in neurologic diseases, neuropsychiatric diseases, and for neurosurgical applications, which may be undetected or otherwise thought to be normal on conventional strengths.

TECHNIQUES

Although the potential of 7-T magnetic resonance (MR) imaging to elucidate novel insights into the pathology of disease has been shown,[1–3] the translation of existing 3-T techniques to higher field strength requires certain considerations. This article introduces the primary tools now used in clinical imaging at 3 T and discusses the underlying physics of the sequences, the primary considerations at 7 T, and recent promising developments using each technique at 7 T.

Gradient Echo

Gradient-echo (GRE) sequences are a versatile class of sequences relying on a GRE generated by the frequency-encoding gradient, which allows transverse dephasing during readout, with contrast coming from the local field inhomogeneity as reflected in dephased protons. The versatility of the GRE sequences comes from their ability to be acquired in two dimensions or three dimensions and to use either single-echo or multiecho gradient refocusing, which allows acquisition of both T2*-weighted magnitude images, as well as images with magnetic susceptibility contrast, such as susceptibility-weighted images (SWI), R2*-mapping, and quantitative susceptibility mapping (QSM), enabling sensitivity to myelin and iron.

Performing GRE imaging at 7 T has been shown to provide enhanced spatial resolution of deep gray structures[4–6] **(Fig. 1)**, enabling better

Funding sources: NIH, PAC-12, GE Healthcare, ASNR.
Funded by: NIH; *Grant number(s):* 1R01AG061120; *NIHMS-ID:* 1631961.
[a] Department of Radiology, Stanford University, 300 Pasteur Drive, Room S047, Stanford, CA 94305-5105, USA;
[b] Division of Neuroradiology, Johns Hopkins University, 600 N. Wolfe St. B-112 D, Baltimore, MD 21287, USA;
[c] Department of Bioengineering, Stanford University, Lucas Center for Imaging, Room P271, 1201 Welch Road, Stanford, CA 94305-5488, USA; [d] Department of Radiology, 300 Pasteur Drive, Room S031, Stanford, CA 94305-5105, USA; [e] Department of Radiology, Stanford University, Lucas Center for Imaging, Room P271, 1201 Welch Road, Stanford, CA 94305-5488, USA
* Corresponding author.
E-mail address: mzeineh@stanford.edu

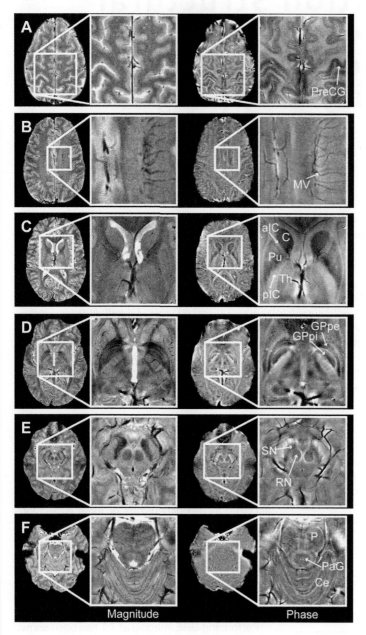

Fig. 1. An example of magnitude and phase imaging contrast at 7 T providing clear visualization of deep gray structures. Magnitude (left) and phase (right) images of the (*A*) precentral gyrus (PreCG), (*B*) medullary veins (MV), (*C*) caudate (C), putamen (Pu), anterior and posterior limbs of the internal capsule (aIC/pIC), thalamus (Th), (*D*) globus pallidus pars interna/pars externa (GPpi/GPpe), (*E*) red nucleus (RN), substantia nigra (SN), (*F*) pons (P), periaqueductal gray matter (PaG), and cerebellum (Ce). (*From* Hammond KE, Lupo JM, Xu D, et al. Development of a robust method for generating 7T multichannel phase images of the brain with application to normal volunteers and patients with neurological diseases. Neuroimage. 2008 Feb 15; 39(4): 1682–1692;with permission.)

segmentation and characterization of normal anatomy and disorder. High-resolution GRE at 7 T has generally been performed with three-dimensional (3D) sequences to maintain high signal/noise ratio (SNR) by exciting an entire imaging volume for each readout, but recent work has developed a novel two-dimensional (2D) simultaneous multislice sequence to serve as an alternative, with the added benefit of higher image contrast and sensitivity to lesions in multiple sclerosis (**Fig. 2**).[7]

QSM uses the frequency shift in the MR imaging signal to map the magnetic field profile within the tissue to determine the spatial distribution of the underlying magnetic susceptibility by solving an inverse problem using the known point spread function of a magnetic dipole.[8,9] Because susceptibility contrast scales with the magnetic field strength, it provides an opportunity to perform higher-resolution susceptibility contrast imaging with higher sensitivity to myelin and iron (**Fig. 3**).[10] Likewise, recent work using 7 T has shown the potential to reduce scan time[11] and provide higher-resolution imaging than at 3 T,[12] which may facilitate better delineation of deep

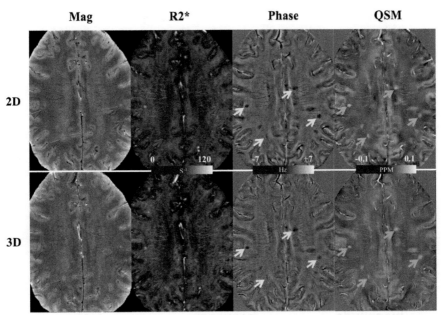

	Mag	R2*	Phase	QSM
2D				
3D				

Fig. 2. Images from the 2D SMS GRE (*top row*) and 3D gradient-echo imaging (*bottom row*) showing improved lesion detection in the 2D magnitude images and comparable detection in R2*, phase, and QSM images of a patient with multiple sclerosis. Overall multiple sclerosis lesions (*arrows*) are visualized almost equally on the R2* (*red arrows*), phase (*yellow arrows*) and QSM (*green arrows*) images. On the magnitude images, 2 lesions (*orange arrows*) have similar visibility, whereas the other 2 (*orange arrowhead*) are better visualized on the 2D image. In addition, the 2D magnitude image shows a sharper edge between gray and white matter. (*From* Bian W, Kerr AB, Tranvinh E, Parivash E, et al. MR susceptibility contrast imaging using a 2D simultaneous multi-slice gradient-echo sequence at 7T. PLoS One. 2019; 14(7); with permission.)

gray matter structures for neurosurgical applications[10] and higher-resolution angiography (**Fig. 4**),[12] enhanced grading of brain tumors,[13] and improved lesion characterization in multiple sclerosis (**Fig. 5**).[14]

Fast Spin Echo

Fast spin echo (FSE) imaging, or turbo spin echo (TSE), uses several refocusing radiofrequency (RF) pulses delivered during each repetition time (TR) interval with a phase-encoding gradient briefly switched on between echoes to allow fast scan times. With high SNR and good contrast, it is a workhorse in clinical imaging at all field strengths. However, FSE is susceptible to B1 inhomogeneities, which are amplified at 7 T because of the shortened wavelength of RF pulses at 7 T and can result in signal loss (**Fig. 6**).[15] In addition, FSE is limited by RF power deposition, which becomes significantly exacerbated at 7 T. However, given the short scan times and the potential to enable high-resolution T2 mapping[16] to discern fine anatomic detail in diseases such as hippocampal subfields in Alzheimer disease[7] (AD) (**Fig. 7**), facilitate high-resolution tissue segmentation,[17] and provide

strong gray-white contrast,[18] developing strategies to address these issues of FSE at 7 T is critical. Adiabatic FSE sequences have been developed and have been shown to provide improved image quality compared with traditional FSE in the brain and neck.[19]

T1-weighted volumetric imaging

Magnetization prepared rapid GRE (MPRAGE) sequences, which rely on a nonselective inversion pulse followed by rapidly acquired GREs, allows lower specific absorption rate (SAR) than traditional FSE sequences. In clinical imaging, MPRAGE and variants are used for anatomic imaging given their high gray-white contrast; in research or quantitative clinical studies, they are the standard for performing brain segmentation. Subsequent work has developed accelerated versions[20] to enable more rapid clinical scanning as well as modified versions. MPRAGE shows extensive susceptibility artifact related to inhomogeneous B0, so a variant called MP2RAGE was developed, where 2 images with different inversion times are combined to suppress dependencies of the receive field (**Fig. 8**).[21] MP2RAGE

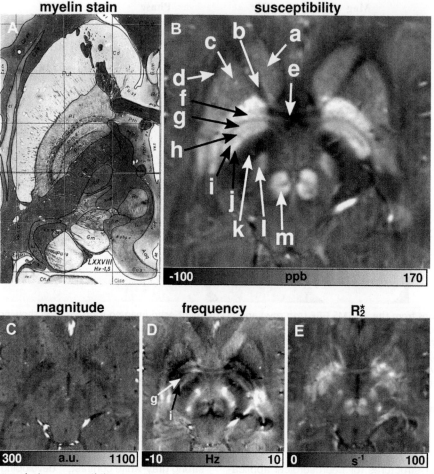

Fig. 3. High-resolution susceptibility imaging compared with myelin stain (*A*). The susceptibility map (*B*) clearly reveals: a, head of the caudate nucleus; b, anterior limb of internal capsule; c, putamen; d, external capsule; e, anterior commissure; f, external globus pallidus; g, lamina pallidi medialis; h, pallidum mediale externum; i, lamina pallidi incompleta; j, pallidum mediale internum; k, posterior limb of internal capsule; l, subthalamic nucleus; m, red nucleus. Quantitative susceptibility mapping (QSM) with magnitude- (*C*), phase-, (*D*) and R2*-imaging (*E*) at ultra-high magnetic field strength are also shown. (*From* Deistung A, Schäfer A, Schweser F, et al. Toward in vivo histology: a comparison of quantitative susceptibility mapping (QSM) with magnitude-, phase-, and R2*-imaging at ultra-high magnetic field strength. Neuroimage. 2013 Jan 15;65:299–314; with permission.)

has been used for T1 structural imaging and morphometry[22,23] as well as whole-brain segmentation.[24] In addition, MPRAGE imaging at 7 T has shown the ability to delineate intracranial vasculature.[25]

The white matter–nulled MPRAGE (WMnMPRAGE) generates additional contrast by suppressing signal from white matter, with inversion times chosen such that fluid is bright, and gray-white contrast is even better than with MPRAGE. This technique is optimized specifically to visualize the thalamus and intrathalamic nuclei (**Fig. 9**).[26] Specifically, it relies on an inversion time close to the white matter-null regime, a lengthened time between successive inversion pulses, and a low flip angle to increase thalamic

signal and contrast.[26] This sequence has been used for automatic thalamic nuclei segmentation to highlight thalamic lesions and improve measurements of thalamic atrophy in patients with multiple sclerosis.[27]

Balanced Steady-state Free Precession

Balanced steady-state free precession (bSSFP) is a variant of GRE in which a steady, residual transverse magnetization is maintained between successive cycles. Gradients are balanced in all axes such that gradient-induced dephasing within TR is exactly zero, offering a very high SNR and relative insensitivity to motion. At 7 T, bSSFP has shown SNR benefits compared with GRE per unit imaging time.[28] Although bSSFP suffers from

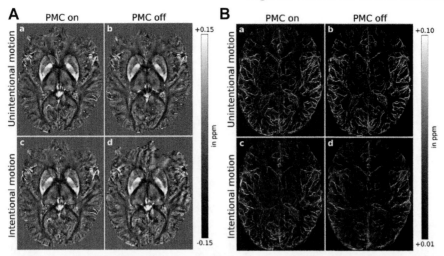

Fig. 4. High-resolution QSM and QSM-based venograms at 7 T. (*Left*) Intrapatient comparison (patient 3) of (A and C) motion-corrected and (B and D) uncorrected QSM, (A and B) without and (C and D) with intentional motion. For small-scale motion, corrected and uncorrected QSM showed no apparent motion artifacts. For large-scale motion, uncorrected maps were degraded; this effect was reduced with motion correction leading to minor residual artifacts. (*Right*) Intrapatient comparison (patient 3) of (A and C) motion-corrected and (B and D) uncorrected QSM-based venograms (A and B) without and (C and D) with intentional motion. For small-scale motion, corrected and uncorrected QSM showed no apparent motion artifacts. Without correction, large-scale motion degraded vessel depiction considerably; this effect was largely prevented by motion correction leading to minor residual artifacts. (*From* Mattern H, Sciarra A, Lüsebrink F, et al. Prospective motion correction improves high-resolution quantitative susceptibility mapping at 7T. Magn Reson Med. 2019 Mar;81(3):1605–1619; with permission.)

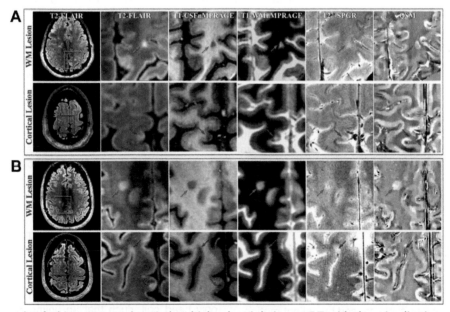

Fig. 5. Example of white matter and cortical multiple sclerosis lesions at 7 T, with clear visualization using QSM. MR images of representative white matter and cortical lesions from patients 4 (*A*) and 5 (*B*). A whole section of the T2 magnetization-prepared fluid-attenuated inversion recovery (FLAIR) image is shown in the left column with a zoomed-in region (*blue/red square*) for all image contrasts. Two white matter lesions (*blue arrows*) and 3 cortical lesions (*red arrows*) are shown. White matter and cortical lesions are hyperintense and hypointense relative to their adjacent parenchyma on QSM images, respectively, whereas both types of lesions show an identical contrast on all other images. CSFnMPRAGE, cerebrospinal fluid–nulled T1-weighted magnetization prepared rapid GRE; WMnMPRAGE, white matter–nulled magnetization prepared rapid GRE. (*From* Bian W, Tranvinh E, Tourdias T, et al. In Vivo 7T MR quantitative susceptibility mapping reveals opposite susceptibility contrast between cortical and white matter lesions in multiple sclerosis. Am J Neuroradiol. 2016;37(10):1808–1815; with permission.)

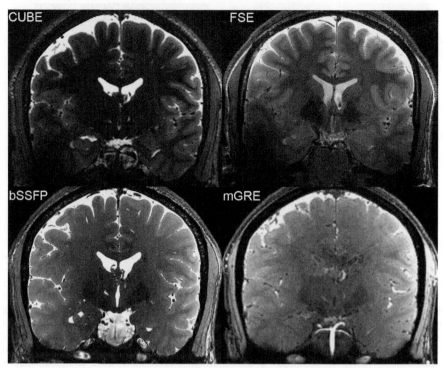

Fig. 6. Relative homogeneity of balanced steady-state free precession (bSSFP) compared with FSE and CUBE. (*From* Zeineh M, Parekh M, Zaharchuk G, et al. Ultrahigh-resolution imaging of the human brain with phase-cycled balanced steady-state free precession at 7 T. Invest Radiol. 2014;49(5):278–289; with permission.)

bands of signal hypointensity caused by B0 inhomogeneity, these can be remedied by phase cycling.[29–31] In addition, bSSFP can be performed with low flip angles to avoid the limitations on SAR that can often be prohibitive at 7 T. bSSFP has a relatively homogeneous signal profile (see **Fig. 6**). These features of bSSFP make it a compelling sequence to use at 7 T and prior work has shown the potential of bSSFP to provide superior anatomic visualization of the hippocampus (**Fig. 10**), cerebellum, and skull base, as well as strong iron contrast.[18,32]

Motion Correction

Despite the promising results of each of these techniques, achieving both high SNR and high resolution at 7 T requires long scan times, which often result in image artifacts caused by patient motion. These motion artifacts limit the clinical interpretability of images and the reliability of quantitative analyses.

Retrospective methods for motion correction are available[33–35] but require longer postprocessing time and may be insufficient, because of overlaps and gaps in k-space.[36] Prospective motion correction can overcome this limitation by using measured head position and orientation to update the imaging volume position and orientation within the bore in real time. The necessary real-time head pose information can be obtained using several techniques, including active markers[37] field probes,[38,39] sequence-navigator-based methods,[40] or optical tracking using a camera system.[41,42] Early optical camera systems relied on multiple cameras external to the bore of the MR imaging scanner,[43,44] making line of sight for long or narrow-bore magnets, enclosed head coils, or large patients a challenge. The development of MR-compatible cameras has made it possible to use cameras within the B0 field of the scanner; for example, attached to the inner surface of the bore or to a rig placed around the receive-only head coil.[42] Prior work at 3 T used a single camera mounted directly on the receive-only head coil, such that an unimpeded view of an optical marker to the patient's head can be achieved between the rungs of the coil.[45,46] However, because most commercial head coils at 7 T are enclosed within an RF transmit shell, reliable line of sight to a head-mounted marker is not possible, leading to the use of mouthpiece-mounted markers that extend beyond the head coil.[47,48] These systems have achieved

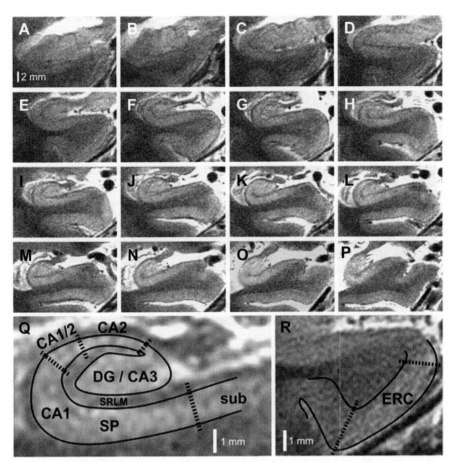

Fig. 7. Substructures of hippocampus and atrophy specific to AD. Hippocampal microstructural imaging at 7 T. (*A–P*) Serial oblique coronal slices, zoomed to the right hippocampus, are shown for 1 of the patients enrolled in this study. Slices are arranged anterior to posterior, using the same scale represented by the bar in panel (*A*). (*Q*) Higher-magnification view of panel (*I*), showing how subfields are demarcated. Areas containing dense collections of neuronal cell bodies (eg, CA1-SP) appear bright on this T2W image, whereas neuropil areas (eg, CA1-SRLM), which contain dense axons, dendrites, myelin, and synapses, appear hypointense. DG, dentate gyrus; CA1–3, cornu ammonis subfields 1 to 3; SP, stratum pyramidale; SRLM, stratum radiatum/stratum lacunosum moleculare; sub, subiculum. (*R*) Higher magnification of the parahippocampal gyrus from (*E*), showing how the entorhinal cortex (ERC) is demarcated. (*From* Bian W, Kerr AB, Tranvinh E, et al. MR susceptibility contrast imaging using a 2D simultaneous multi-slice gradient-echo sequence at 7T. PLoS One. 2019; 14(7); with permission.)

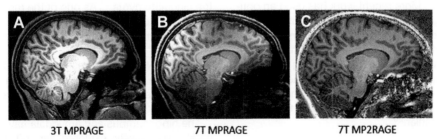

Fig. 8. MPRAGE at 3 T (*A*), 7-T MPRAGE (*B*), and 7-T MP2RAGE (*C*) acquired on a single patient. MPRAGE at 7 T (*B*) shows a strong bias field, giving low signal intensities in temporal and basal regions. The 7-T MP2RAGE sequence (*C*) accounts for this bias field and delivers good contrast properties between gray and white matter more homogeneously throughout the brain, although still with some regions of inhomogeneity inferiorly. (*From* Seiger R, Hahn A, Hummer A, et al. Voxel-based morphometry at ultra-high fields: A comparison of 7T and 3T MRI data. Neuroimage. 2015 Jun; 113: 207–216; with permission.)

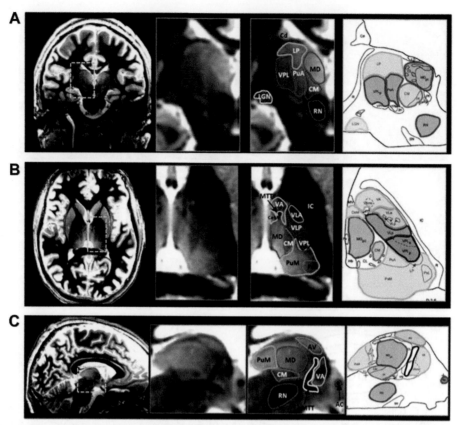

Fig. 9. Representative examples of WMnMPRAGE scans in coronal, axial, and sagittal places (each orientation shown in a different volunteer) and presented with the corresponding histologic plates (Morel and colleagues, 1997[49]). Several nuclei can be identified with the enhanced intrinsic contrast between adjacent structures, particularly with the hypointense bands that isolate structures that are close in signal intensity. For example, see the thin boundaries around the pulvinar anterior (PuA, *green*) in coronal view (*A*), around the ventral anterior nucleus (VA, *pink*) in axial view (*B*), and around the anterior ventral nucleus (AV, *orange*) in sagittal view (*C*). (*From* Tourdias T, Saranathan M, Levesque IR, et al. Visualization of intra-thalamic nuclei with optimized white-matter-nulled MPRAGE at 7T. Neuroimage. 2014;84:534–545; with permission.)

higher-resolution structural imaging in volunteers than would otherwise be achievable (**Fig. 11**)[47] and can provide improved quantitative susceptibility maps.[48] More recent work has used an optical tracking system for 7 T using a custom-built, within-coil camera to track a marker mounted on a patient's forehead, which has shown the ability to perform ultrahigh-resolution imaging of the hippocampus (**Fig. 12**) and may improve accessibility of motion correction during 7-T examinations and enable more robust use of all of the techniques discussed earlier.[50]

ANATOMIC APPLICATIONS
Limbic System

The limbic system is fundamental to emotion, memory, and cognitive function.[51–53] It is composed of multiple structures, including the hippocampus, amygdala, parahippocampal gyrus, mammillary bodies, anterior thalamic nuclei, and the cingulate gyrus.[51] As one of the most intricate circuits in the brain, neuroimaging plays an essential role in understanding the anatomic and functional role of this system in particular. The superior SNR of high-resolution structural 7 T can provide greater detail of the architecture of the structures of this system for clinical applications (**Fig. 13**).[52]

The hippocampus and amygdala have been the most exhaustively explored for 7-T evaluation within the limbic system, providing exquisite detail on these small structures.[52,53] These structures are crucial to memory encoding/retrieval and emotion, respectively, and disorders in these regions can have significant clinical implications.

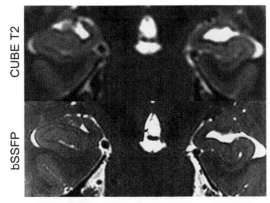

Fig. 10. Improved imaging of the hippocampus using bSSFP compared with CUBE T2. Hippocampal heads in a healthy volunteer in time-matched CUBE T2 (*top*) and bSSFP (*bottom*). The left-right asymmetry is caused by a slight head rotation. (*From* Zeineh M, Parekh M, Zaharchuk G, et al. Ultrahigh-resolution imaging of the human brain with phase-cycled balanced steady-state free precession at 7 T. Invest Radiol. 2014;49(5):278–289; with permission.)

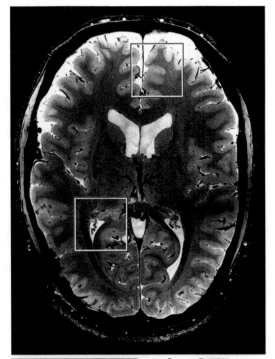

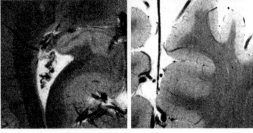

Fig. 11. Single slice high-resolution GRE scan enabled by motion correction. At a resolution of 0.12 × 0.12 × 0.6 mm, structures of 1 to 2 pixels in width are identifiable and clearly defined. Magnifications of the marked regions are shown below. (*From* Stucht D, Danishad KA, Schulze P, et al. Highest Resolution In Vivo Human Brain MRI Using Prospective Motion Correction. PLoS One. 2015;10(7); with permission.)

The basic hippocampal subfields are the dentate gyrus (DG), cornu ammonis 1 to 4 (CA1–CA4), subiculum (SUB), and entorhinal and perirhinal cortices, as well as the key white matter pathways such as the fornix (starting at alveus, then the fimbria, and finally the fornix) and parahippocampal gyrus (PHG) (**Fig. 14**).[53] Given that these structures are small and tightly interpositioned, 7 T better delineates these structures with improved resolution compared with 3 T. This difference could be particularly helpful in the hippocampal head, which is extensively folded.[54,55] One reason is that the improved SNR allows higher-resolution imaging. In addition, the increased susceptibility corresponding with the deoxyhemoglobin within the veins creates shorter T2* weighting of the surrounding tissues, which, in turn, increases contrast resolution.[53] This technique also allows visualization of submillimeter venous structures, which are not detectable on 3 T.[53]

Although the basic hippocampal units can be seen on 3 T, 7 T provides a greater understanding of the subfield anatomy. Zeineh and colleagues[18] elucidated the hippocampal subfield architecture on balanced steady-state free precession (bSSFP), where, at ultrahigh resolution, they further showed the appearance of the striatum radiatum and lacunosum moleculare (SRLM), which corresponded with the hypointense T2 band seen within CA1 (**Fig. 15**).[18] Parekh and colleagues[32] used a similar approach by segmenting the white matter pathways involving the

hippocampus, with special attention to the hilus and the previously invisible endfolial pathway, which was validated histologically and expanded on through ex vivo polarized light microscopy.[32,55] Wisse and colleagues[3,56] delineated the hippocampal subfield architecture through automated segmentation of CA1, DG, and SUB in order to achieve an easy, applicable protocol.[56]

In addition to the hippocampus, the amygdala has also been explored on high-resolution 7-T acquisition. The amygdala contains many nuclei, which are connected to the prefrontal cortex,

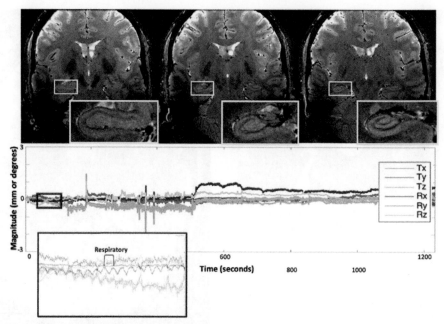

Fig. 12. High-resolution imaging of hippocampus enabled by prospective motion correction. Results of the 20-minute ultrahigh-resolution 2D GRE sequence, showing exquisite imaging quality of the hippocampus and the remainder of the visualized brain. The plots below each image show the translational and rotational motion across time, with the vertical axis showing millimeters and degrees of displacement or rotation, respectively, and the horizontal axis showing time in seconds. Each direction of motion was normalized to the patient's initial position for this scan to visualize only net motion during the acquisition. The purple and orange insets show detection of physiologic respiratory motion, respectively, in addition to rigid-head motion. (*From* DiGiacomo P, Maclaren J, Aksoy M, et al. A within-coil optical prospective motion-correction system for brain imaging at 7T. Magn Reson Med. 2020 Sep;84(3):1661–1671; with permission.)

insula, and thalami in addition to other parts of the limbic system, where it plays a major role in emotional processing, particularly with fear and anxiety.[57] On 3 T, some of these nuclei, such as the medial, lateral, and basolateral ventral medial nuclei, can be faintly separated, although not nearly as well as on pathology.[58] However, as with other structures, 7 T provides superior anatomic detail (see **Fig. 13**).[57]

Given the close anatomic relationship between the hippocampus and amygdala and their synergistic function with emotion and memory, the amygdalohippocampal border (AHB) has also become an area of interest. Derix and colleagues[52] explored the AHB on 7 T and found better delineation and improved contrast of the shape and extent of the alveus, which comprises most of the AHB, on T1-weighted (T1W) imaging, compared with 3 T.

Alzheimer disease

AD is the most common type of neurodegenerative disease and is thought to be caused by accumulation of cortical amyloid plaque and neurofibrillary tangle deposition leading to progressive and unrelenting dementia.[1,59] High-resolution 7 T in the limbic system, compared with 3 T, has made several advancements in the understanding of neurodegenerative diseases and has the potential to improve timely diagnosis and management.[1]

Evaluation at 3 T has been exhaustively explored, providing some insights on neuroanatomical abnormalities in AD, particularly within the hippocampus. These 3-T studies have shown a characteristic atrophy pattern in AD with thinning of the entorhinal cortex (ERC).[60] With the increased SNR at 7 T, the extent and detail of this ERC thinning has been further investigated. In multiple studies, Kerchner and colleagues[1,61–63] reported atrophy in CA1, which includes the SRLM, as well as the ERC in patients with AD, and also showed correlation with delayed recall performance (see **Fig. 7**). Subsequently, the investigators found that the CA1-SRLM atrophy was disproportionately seen in patients with the APOE-e4 allele.[1,61–63]

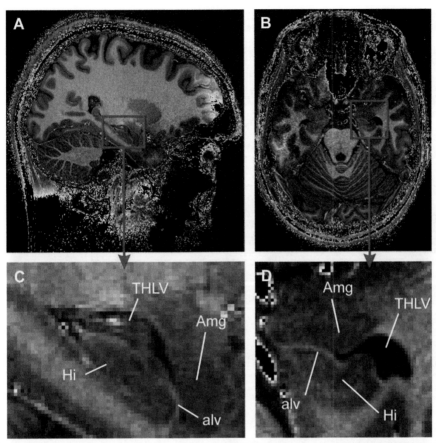

Fig. 13. The increased anatomic detail of the anteromedial temporal lobe on 7-T MPRAGE (divided by a short-echo-time GRE for better signal homogeneity) compared with 3 T. The amygdala (Amg) and the hippocampus (Hi) are seen in the mediotemporal lobe of S1. (*A*) T1-weighted in vivo MR imaging in the sagittal plane. The amygdalohippocampal area, marked by a red square, is magnified in (*C*). The corresponding axial view is shown in (*B*) and the magnified amygdalo-hippocampal border area is shown in (*D*). The border between the amygdala and the hippocampus formed by the temporal horn of the lateral ventricle (THLV) and the alveus (alv) can be clearly seen. (*From* Derix J, Yang S, Lüsebrink F, et al. Visualization of the amygdalo–hippocampal border and its structural variability by 7T and 3T magnetic resonance imaging. Human Brain Mapping. 2014 March 12; 35(9): p. 4316–4329; with permission.)

Other groups have also corroborated the EC's role within AD on high-resolution 7-T evaluation. Tangle deposition occurs early within the ERC, which is a part of the anterior PHG and is affected in early preclinical stages of AD.[64] Wisse and colleagues[65] also used 7 T to evaluate AD in early stages where they found volume loss in multiple subfields, including CA1, SUB, CA4, and DG in 17 patients. Similarly, Boutet and colleagues[66] assessed differences in hippocampal subfield volume on 7 T, showing reduction in CA1-3 and SUB in 11 patients.

In addition to morphometric analyses of the hippocampal subfields, high-resolution 7 T has allowed further exploration of AD, and neurodegenerative diseases in general, on other conventional sequences. T2* imaging on 7 T was also used by van Rooden and colleagues[67] in a 16-patient cohort, where they found increased phase shift within the frontal, temporal, and parietal cortices corresponding with regions of amyloid plaque deposition (**Fig. 16**). High-resolution 7 T has also elucidated other potential radiological-pathologic correlations. Zeineh and colleagues[68] identified T2* hypointensities within the subiculum in patients with AD on high-resolution ex vivo 7-T evaluation, showing the role of microglia-mediated iron deposition as opposed to tau or amyloid deposition. Other ex vivo explorations that may be translated to human imaging include that of Kenkhuis and colleagues,[69] who also used T2* on 7 T where

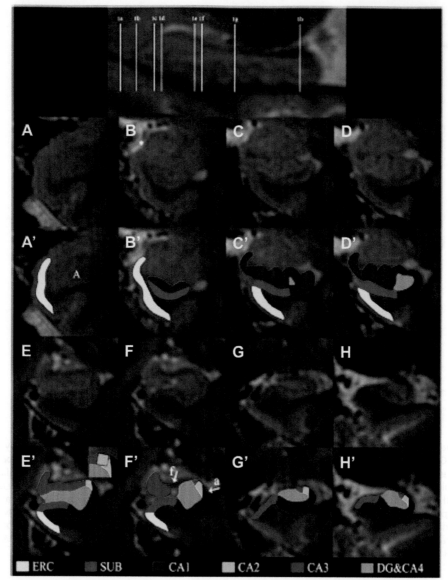

Fig. 14. Highlighted subfields of the hippocampal formation at 7-T 3D T2-weighted (T2W) FSE. The upper figure shows a sagittal view with references to all the coronal images. Coronal images of the hippocampal formation are shown in A–H in an anterior-to-posterior direction. The head is shown in B–F, the body in G, and the tail in H. The asterisk in B indicates the sulcus semiannularis. The segmentation of the hippocampal formation is shown in A′–H′. The zoom-in in E′ shows the construction of the border between CA2 and CA3 by drawing a virtual square. The arrows in F point to the alveus and fimbria, which were excluded from segmentation. These hypointense structures are also visible on E′, G′, and H′. (*From* Wisse L E M, Gerritsen L, Zwanenburg JJM, et al. Subfields of the hippocampal formation at 7T MRI: In vivo volumetric assessment. Neuroimage. 2012;61(4):1043–1049; with permission.)

they showed cortical lamination disruption in AD, especially in advanced stages, within the temporal and fusiform gyri in addition to overall severe atrophy (**Fig. 17**).

Epilepsy Evaluation at 7 T has also aided in the understanding of other disorders that affect the hippocampus, namely entities causing epilepsy.

Approximately 60% of patients with epilepsy are symptomatic because of a localized lesion,[70] with hippocampal sclerosis (HS)[71] and focal cortical dysplasia[70] being some of the more common entities. Evaluation at 3 T is most widely used for identifying a localized epileptogenic focus, but some studies show a low detection rate of 26%,[72] which can have far-reaching consequences for

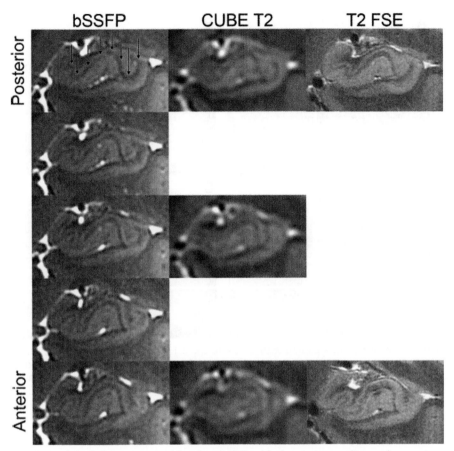

Fig. 15. Comparison of the left hippocampal head on bSSFP with the stratum radiatum, lacunosum, and molec-ulare highlighted (*black arrows*). CUBE T2 and T2 FSE images are also shown in native space without interpola-tion. (*From* Zeineh M, Parekh M, Zaharchuk G, et al. Ultrahigh-resolution imaging of the human brain with phase-cycled balanced steady-state free precession at 7 T. Invest Radiol. 2014;49(5):278–289; with permission.)

such patients because they are less likely to un-dergo surgery and, in the event that they do, because of the incompletely localization, this epileptogenic focus is missed or incompletely resected.[73] In contrast, 7 T, with its exquisite anatomic details, has been shown in several studies to improve detection and overall under-standing of epileptogenic foci.[2] In doing so, 7 T could aid not only in lesion detection but also in presurgical planning.[74]

Increases in field strength have shown improved localized lesion detection in epilepsy. At clinical strengths, 3 T is superior to 1.5 T at detecting new lesions as well as improving visualization of known lesions.[75] Many studies have focused on improved detection of lesions on 7 T with previ-ously normal examinations on clinical strengths. For instance, in patients with normal conventional 3-T or 1.5-T MR imaging, in a 21-patient cohort, De Ciantis and colleagues[76] reported that 7-T GRE and fluid-attenuated inversion recovery

(FLAIR) sequences detected localized structural abnormalities in 29% of these patients, all of which were deemed unremarkable at 3 T. Four of these 6 patients were found to have pathology-proven focal cortical dysplasia on resection (**Fig. 18**). Examples of such lesions include hippocampal abnormalities, polymicrogyria, and cortical irregu-larities.[76] Other studies have also shown similar re-sults in the superiority of 7 T in lesional detection compared with 3 T.[73,77]

Several studies have also shown superior detail or increased diagnostic confidence of known localized epileptogenic lesions on 7 T compared with 3 T. Feldman and colleagues[78] showed superior visualization of asymmetric perivascular spaces in patients with focal epi-lepsy. A previous study also reported increased diagnostic confidence of multiple disorders, including epileptogenic foci, with interrater agreement of 93.3% on 7 T compared with 69.7% on 3 T (**Fig. 19**).[79]

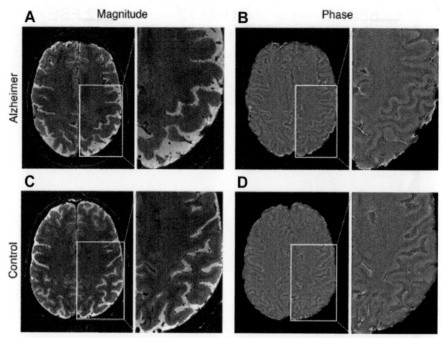

Fig. 16. Axial 2D GRE images show a patient with AD (*A, B*) and a 1 normal control patient (*C, D*). (*A, C*) Magnitude images. (*B, D*) Phase images. The phase images show the enhanced contrast between gray and white matter in the patient with AD compared with the control patient, as indicated by the larger cortical phase shift. (*From* van Rooden S, Versluis MJ, Liem MJ, et al. Cortical phase changes in Alzheimer's disease at 7T MRI: a novel imaging marker. Alzheimers Dement. 2014 Jan;10(1):e19–26; with permission.)

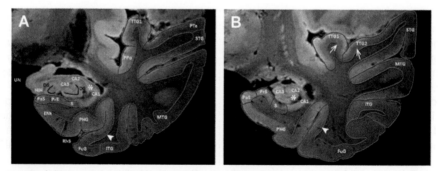

Fig. 17. Contours of the anterior hippocampus and midhippocampus on coronal plane on 7-T T1W ex vivo imaging. Control brain segmented for the areas of interest in 2 coronal planes showing the hippocampus anterior and mid; medial temporal lobe subregions were segmented based on contours of the sulci and gyri and signal intensity of cortical lamination on MR imaging. Contrast appears similar to T2W images because of formalin fixation. Hyperintense band of CA3, CA2, and CA1 (*asterisk, A, B*). Thin band of Baillarger (*arrowhead, A, B*). Broad band of Baillarger (*open arrows, B*). TTG1, anterior transverse temporal gyrus; CA1/2/3, cornu ammonis 1/2/3 substructures of the hippocampus; DG, dentate gyrus; ERC, entorhinal cortex; FD, fascia dentate; FuG, fusiform gyrus; HiH, hippocampal head; ITG, inferior temporal gyrus; MTG, middle temporal gyrus; PHG, parahippocampal gyrus; PaS, parasubiculum; PPo, planum polare; Pte, planum temporale; TTG2, posterior transverse temporal gyrus; PrS, presubiculum; RhS, rhinal sulcus; S, subiculum; STG, superior temporal gyrus; UN, uncus. (*From* Kenkhuis B, Jonkman LE, Bulk M, et al. 7T MRI allows detection of disturbed cortical lamination of the medial temporal lobe in patients with Alzheimer's disease. Neuroimage Clin. 2019;21:101665; with permission.)

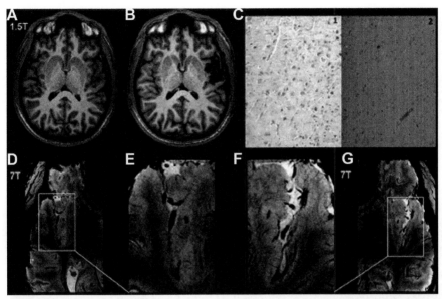

Fig. 18. A patient with intractable epilepsy evaluated at 1.5 and 7 T. Preoperative 3D SPGR at 1.5 T (*A*); 1.5-T postoperative 3D SPGR (*B*); histopathology (*C*); 7-T 2D GRE, right hemisphere (*D*); magnification of (*D*) (*E*); 7-T axial 3D GRE (*F*); magnification of (*F*) (*G*). (*A, D,* and *E*) No structural abnormalities. (*B*) Postoperative MR imaging showing the extent of resection. (*C*) Histologic section showing cortical laminar disruption and dysmorphic neurons, consistent with FCD IIa. Of note, (*D*) and its magnified image (*E*) show normal distinction between white and gray matter in the right superior temporal gyrus and the insula. In contrast, (*G*) and its magnified image (*F*) show blurring of the gray-white matter junction in the anterior part of the left superior temporal gyrus and in the insular gyri (*C1*, Kluver stain, original magnification ×200; *C2*, hematoxylin-eosin, original magnification ×100). (*From* De Ciantis A, Barba C, Tassi L, et al. 7T MRI in focal epilepsy with unrevealing conventional field strength imaging. Epilepsia. 2016 Mar;57(3):445–54; with permission.)

HS is 1 such example of a detectable epileptogenic focus. Initially, Breyer and colleagues[71] showed the utility of 7 T in detecting HS, which was confirmed in their pilot study with 6 patients.[71,74] Additional studies have further elucidated the role of the hippocampal architecture in epilepsy. For example, Stefanits and colleagues[80] showed the clinical feasibility of 7 T in detecting HS, where they found a sensitivity and specificity of 100%. Gillman and colleagues[81] expanded on this histologic correlation by showing that HS subtypes can be distinguished on 7-T evaluation in their ex vivo analysis. Voets and colleagues[82] then extended this morphometric evaluation in reexamining clinically normal MR scans, which were initially scanned on either 1.5 or 3 T. On reexamination on 7 T with MR spectroscopy (MRS), they found hippocampal subfield atrophy, mostly affecting CA3, in 75% of the patients. They also found that SUB atrophy correlated with verbal memory dysfunction. In addition, they also reported decreased glutamine levels in most of these patients, which was also implicated in decreased verbal memory performance.[82]

Midbrain

Anatomy

The midbrain is affected in several disease entities, such as neuropsychiatric and neurodegenerative motor diseases. The intricate anatomy of the midbrain has been crucial in the understanding of these disorders, particularly with respect to the dopaminergic system, mainly comprising the substantia nigra (SN) and the ventral tegmental area (VTA).[83] This system has been specifically implicated in reward, motivation, and attention, among other functions.[83] However, most of the current work has been performed on clinical magnet strengths (either 1.5 or 3 T), which has provided some anatomic detail, but the greater resolution on 7 T has expanded knowledge of the anatomy.[83]

Several relevant midbrain structures can be visualized on clinical strengths, including the SN, VTA, and the red nucleus (RN). At present, on

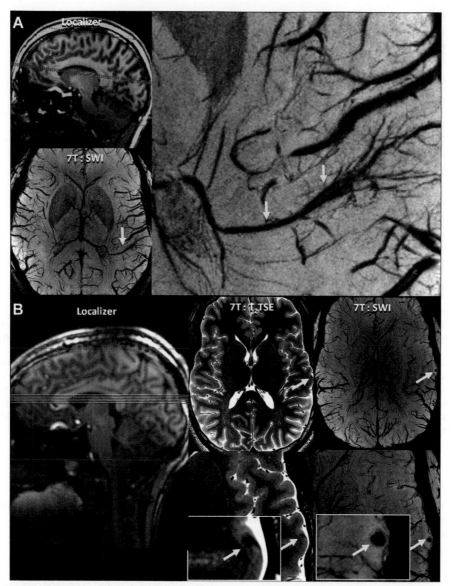

Fig. 19. Lesions identified on SWI. (*A*) Patient 17, clockwise from top left: localizer image showing the location of the axial slices; an enlarged view of a developmental venous anomaly (DVA) associated with the suspected seizure onset zone identified on the SWI; full axial slice of 7-T SWI minimum intensity projection showing a DVA.(*B*) Patient 10, left to right: localizer image showing the location of the axial slices; T2 TSE slice (full slice above, enlarged image below) showing a cortical thickness defect indicated by a yellow arrow, initially identified on SWI; SWI slice (full slice above, enlarged image below) showing a punctate focus of susceptibility indicated by a yellow arrow colocalized with a cortical thickness defect. (*From* Feldman RE, Delman BN, Pawha PS, et al. 7T MRI in epilepsy patients with previously normal clinical MRI exams compared against healthy controls. PLoS One. 2019;14(3); with permission.)

such strengths, the SN can be delineated into its subparts on clinical T2-weighted (T2W) imaging, where the medial and lateral aspects represent the pars reticulata (SNr) and pars compacta (SNc).[2,84] However, the small inner structures of the SN, and VTA, cannot be seen on these strengths.[2] Many of these small structures contain neuromelanin or iron, which allows increased visualization, delineation, and quantification on higher-resolution 7 T, most notably on SWI and QSM (**see Fig. 4; Figs. 20** and **21**).[2] The vascularization of these structures, particularly in the SN and RN, is also difficult to visualize on clinical strengths, and is another area where 7 T provides more anatomic

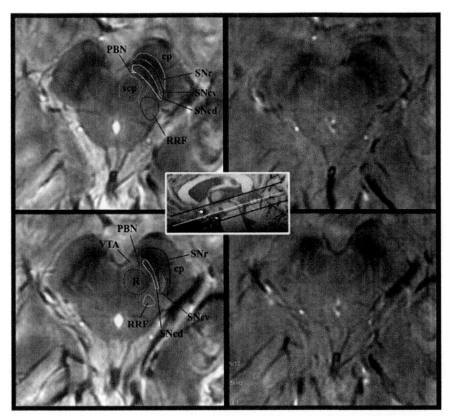

Fig. 20. Susceptibility weighted angiography (SWAN)-targeted axial image of the midbrain in a healthy patient evaluated at 3 T (*right column*) and at 7 T (*left column*). The trilaminar organization of the SN at level II (*upper row*) and the nigrosome formation at level I (*lower row*) are clearly shown with 3-T and 7-T magnets. Levels I and II of image acquisition are represented by white and gray lines in the scout image. On 7-T images, we overlaid a diagram of the trilaminar structure of the SN derived by anatomic atlases.[41] The diagnostic accuracy is increased for both high-field-strength and ultrahigh-field-strength magnets. Cp, cerebral peduncle; PBN, parabrachial nucleus; R, red nucleus; RRF, retrorubral field; scp, superior cerebellar peduncle; SNcv, substantia nigra pars compacta ventralis; SNcd, substantia nigra pars compacta dorsalis; SNr, substantia nigra pars reticularis. (*From* Cosottini M, Frosini D, Pesaresi I, et al. Comparison of 3T and 7T susceptibility-weighted angiography of the substantia nigra in diagnosing Parkinson disease. AJNR Am J Neuroradiol. 2015 Mar;36(3):461–6; with permission.)

details.[83] Eapen and colleagues[83] showed that the boundaries, substructure, and different vascularization patterns of the SN, VTA, and RN were more distinctly visible on T2W and T2*W sequences on 7 T (**Fig. 22**).

Parkinson disease

High-resolution 7 T has shown promise in neurogenerative diseases affecting the midbrain, such as Parkinson disease (PD). Dysfunction within the previously detailed dopaminergic pathway manifests as symptoms of PD, specifically involving the SN. With the lower SNR and contrast resolution, clinical field strengths are insufficient in definitively delineating inner structures of the SN for diagnosis of PD.[85] Identification of the central hyperintense component in the lateral aspect of the normal mid-SN, for example, is less certain

on 3 T.[2] Although the lower SNR decreases accuracy, 3 T can still have utility in identifying true-negative studies with high specificity.[2] However, on 7 T, the 3-layer organizational structure of the SN, specifically the iron-containing components, can be more readily distinguished, allowing improved accuracy in diagnosis and follow-up.[85] For instance, 1 such abnormal finding in which 7 T has superior accuracy compared with 3 T is the loss of nigrosome 1 within the SN, which is an iron-containing inner structure. Cosottini and colleagues[85] specifically showed that 7 T is highly accurate in detecting normal-appearing SNs in patients without PD and SN abnormalities in patients with known PD (**Fig. 23**). In a subsequent study by the same group, they found higher accuracy of true-positive cases of PD on 7 T compared with 3 T on SWI.[2] They concluded that 3 T is sufficient

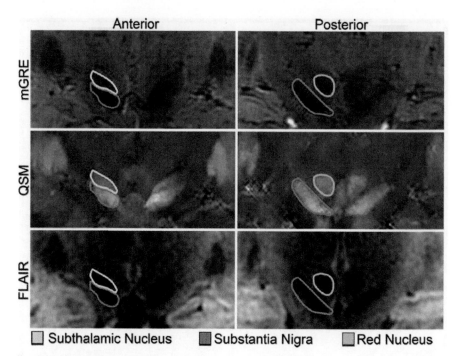

Fig. 21. Midbrain nuclei segmentation. Coronal images of the STN, SN, and RN on multi-echo gradient echo (*top*), QSM (*middle*), and FLAIR (*bottom*). (*From* Poston KL, Ua Cruadhlaoich MAI, Santoso LF, et al. Substantia Nigra Volume Dissociates Bradykinesia and Rigidity from Tremor in Parkinson's Disease: A 7 Tesla Imaging Study. J Parkinsons Dis. 2020;10(2):591–604; with permission.)

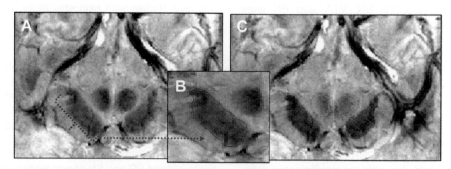

Fig. 22. (*A*) Sample segmented section in the midbrain in both hybride echo sequence and gradient echo sequence scans at the level of the mammillary bodies. (*B*) Segmented SN traced in red in the midbrain. (*C*) Segmented structures (SN is red; VTA, blue; and RN, green) overlaid on the anatomic steady state gradient echo image. (*From* Eapen M, Zald DH, Gatenby JC, et al. Using high-resolution MR imaging at 7T to evaluate the anatomy of the midbrain dopaminergic system. Am J Neuroradiol. 2011;32(4):688–694; with permission.)

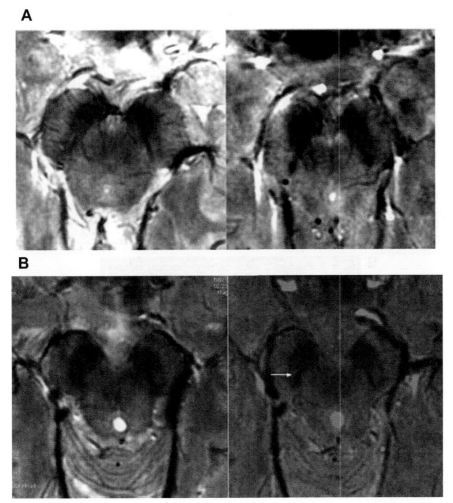

Fig. 23. (*Top, A*) Axial SWAN images in a normal healthy patient at the midbrain at 7 T (*left*) and 3 T (*right*) show visualization of the nigrosome complex on 7 T but this is lost at 3 T (false-positive). (*Bottom, B*) Axial SWAN images in a patient with Parkinson disease at 7 T (*left*) and 3 T (*right*) showing loss of the nigrosome formation on 7 T, whereas the hyperintense band (*white arrow*) was erroneously interpreted as nigrosome (false-negative). (*From* Cosottini M, Frosini D, Pesaresi I, et al. Comparison of 3T and 7T susceptibility-weighted angiography of the substantia nigra in diagnosing Parkinson disease. AJNR Am J Neuroradiol. 2015 Mar;36(3):461–6; with permission.)

for clinical practice given the high specificity. However, in patients with high probability of PD with negative imaging on 3 T, 7 T would be warranted.[2]

SN volume is also an important characteristic within PD. Poston and colleagues[86] correlated SN atrophy with longer disease duration as well as both bradykinesia and rigidity, thus showing that SN volume could serve as a potential biomarker in diagnosis and prognosis of PD.

Major Depressive Disorder

High-resolution 7 T has made progress in neuropsychiatric disorders as well, where early detection can also improve both diagnosis and prognosis. Of the neuropsychiatric disorders, major depressive disorder (MDD), which is characterized by loss of pleasure (anhedonia); lack of concentration; appetite, sleep, and memory disturbances; hopelessness; and so forth, is one of the most common, with 1 in 6 adults affected.[87,88]

Studies on clinical strengths have shown anatomic abnormalities in patients with MDD, with the amygdala, hippocampus, and insula being most affected.[88] As previously discussed in detail, the SNR on 7 T allows greater anatomic visualization of the amygdala, hippocampus, and their inner structures. This property has been especially relevant on 7 T because studies have found more accurate volumetric evaluation of these regions in correlation with MDD symptoms. Brown and colleagues,[87] specifically, performed

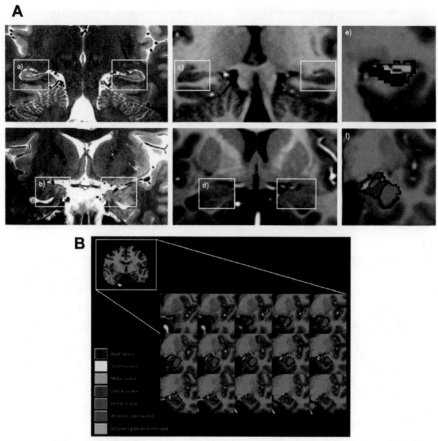

Fig. 24. (*Top*) T2W coronal images of the hippocampal head and amygdala (*A, B*) with corresponding T1W coronal images (*C, D*). Segmented hippocampal and amygdala nuclei (*E, F*). (*Bottom*) Anatomic representation of the segmented amygdala nuclei. (*From* Brown SG, Rutland JW, Verma G, et al. Structural MRI at 7T reveals amygdala nuclei and hippocampal subfield volumetric association with Major Depressive Disorder symptom severity. Sci Rep. 2019;9(1):1–10; with permission.)

a volumetric evaluation of the limbic system and correlated their findings to MDD symptom severity, and they found volume reduction of the amygdala corresponds to increased MDD symptomatic severity (**Fig. 24**).

Although classically the limbic system is affected in MDD, recent studies have also identified circuitry disturbances involving the VTA of the midbrain.[89] At clinical strengths, the VTA is difficult to delineate.[89] However, Morris and colleagues[89] reported that the increased temporal SNR on 7 T allows improved visualization of the several implicated brain regions, including the VTA. Specifically on 7 T, they found hyperconnectivity between the VTA and anterior cingulate cortex, consistent with early findings of MDD

(**Fig. 25**). These findings were not detected on 3 T.[89]

THALAMUS
Anatomy

The thalamus and its adjacent structures, such as the subthalamus and epithalamus, play important roles as relay centers within the brain, transmitting both sensory and motor signals between different regions.[90] The diencephalon consists of the thalamus, epithalamus (which includes the habenula), hypothalamus, and subthalamus. These clusters are important, serving as the focal points of signal transmission, and have been implicated in several disease processes, such as PD, essential tremor (ET) schizophrenia, and MDD.[90] Therefore,

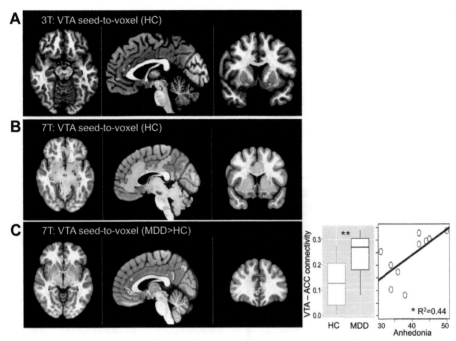

Fig. 25. Connectivity of the VTA with whole brain is shown for 3 T (*A*) and 7 T (*B*) in healthy controls (HC) (voxelwise *P*<.001 for illustration). (*C*) VTA-to-whole-brain functional connectivity comparison between patients with MDD and HC (*P*<.01 voxelwise, cluster>200). Seed-to-seed VTA-anterior cingulate cortex connectivity is plotted for MDD and HC and against anhedonia in the MDD group. (*From* Morris LS, Kundu P, Costi S, et al. Ultra-high field MRI reveals mood-related circuit disturbances in depression: a comparison between 3-Tesla and 7-Tesla. Transl Psychiatry. 2019;9(1):94; with permission.)

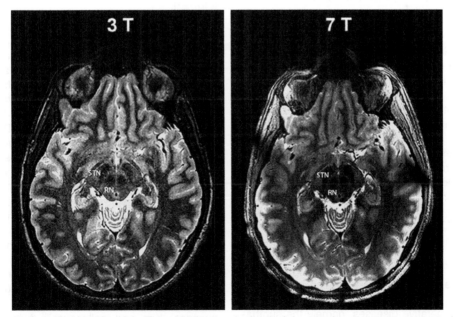

Fig. 26. Both 3-T (*left*) and 7-T (*right*) T2W evaluation at the level of the STN showing more anatomic distinction on 7 T. (*From* Abasch A, Yacoub E, Ugurbil K, et al. An assessment of current brain targets for deep brain stimulation surgery with susceptibility-weighted imaging at 7 tesla. Neurosurgery. 2010;67(6):1745–1756; with permission.)

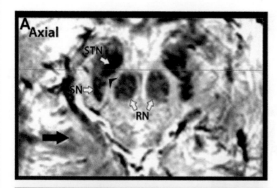

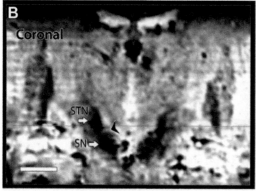

Fig. 27. Axial (*top, A*) and coronal (*bottom, B*) SWI images on 7 T showing distinction boundaries between the STN and SN. (*From* Abasch A, Yacoub E, Ugurbil K, et al. An assessment of current brain targets for deep brain stimulation surgery with susceptibility-weighted imaging at 7 tesla. Neurosurgery. 2010;67(6):1745–1756; with permission.)

accurate identification of these substructures is crucial for neuroanatomical mapping and potential neurosurgical intervention.

Several thalamic and epithalamic nuclei have been identified and have been shown to play critical roles in disease processes. However, clinical strengths are insufficient for accurate targeting. Internal references, such as the anterior and posterior commissures, are currently necessary for more precise localization in these cases. With the higher SNR and increased contrast, high-resolution 7 T has shown great promise in delineation of these small thalamic substructures without the need for internal references, particular on WMnMPRAGE sequences (see **Fig. 9**).[5,26,91] Although many of these substructures have been identified, the focus in this article is on the clinical relevant nuclei implicated in neurodegenerative diseases, namely the subthalamic nucleus (STN) and ventral thalamic nuclei, as well as the epithalamic nuclei in neuropsychiatric disease.

Movement Disorders

Movement disorders, such as PD, can benefit from invasive procedures such as deep brain stimulation (DBS) that target specific nuclei.[92] In order to both maximize efficacy and minimize unnecessary complications, these procedures require precise anatomic localization of the target regions within the thalamus.[92] The STN, which is a motor nucleus ventral to the thalamus, is the most frequent target in DBS for movement disorders.[5,92,93] The STN, in particular, cannot be adequately differentiated from the SN on clinical strengths, but can be distinguished on 7 T (see **Fig. 21; Fig. 26**).[5] One group reported that the increased contrast allowed definitive delineation of the STN from the SN on 7-T SWI in a small cohort (**Fig. 27**).[5] Similar findings were also shown in prior animal studies.[94]

In addition to PD, drug-resistant ET is a movement disorder that benefits from invasive procedures such as DBS or other forms of stereotactic radiosurgery.[92] In such cases, the ventrointermediate nucleus (Vim), which primarily relays motor information from the thalamus to the basal ganglia and motor cortex, is often the target.[92] However, this small nucleus cannot be adequately visualized on clinical strengths, necessitating the use of adjacent anatomic landmarks, such as the quadrilatere of Guiot.[92] However, multiple studies have shown the value of 7 T in definitive delineation of the Vim (**Fig. 28**).[92,93]

Neuropsychiatric Disorders

The habenula, which is part of the epithalamus and adjacent to the dorsomedial thalamus, is an important structure previously implicated in MDD and addiction as a part of the reward pathway.[95] The lateral habenula, which receives input from the basal ganglia and is overactivated in MDD, is often targeted for DBS in order to treat drug-resistant patients with MDD.[96] However, because of the small size, the habenula is difficult to delineate on clinical-strength magnets, making it challenging for patients in whom DBS is warranted.[95,96] The increased SNR and contrast that 7 T provides allow better delineation of these epithalamic nuclei within the habenula. For example, Strotmann and colleagues[95] reported that the medial and lateral habenula were reliably distinguished on 7 T using diffusion-weighted imaging and convention T1W, T2W, and GRE sequences. Kim and colleagues[96] furthered this analysis in a segmentation comparison of the habenular boundaries and volumes on 3 T and 7 T. They determined that the habenular

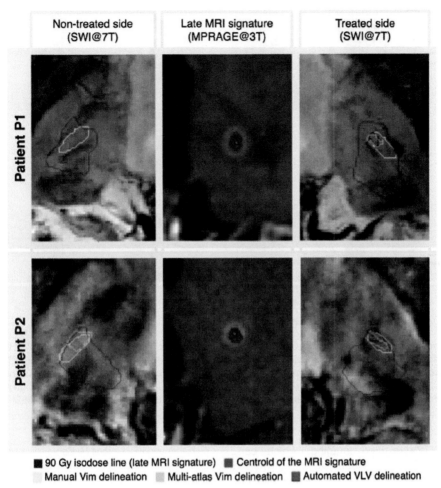

| Non-treated side (SWI@7T) | Late MRI signature (MPRAGE@3T) | Treated side (SWI@7T) |

■ 90 Gy isodose line (late MRI signature)   ■ Centroid of the MRI signature
Manual Vim delineation   Multi-atlas Vim delineation   ■ Automated VLV delineation

Fig. 28. Patients with tremor. Both were treated with the left thalamus with left Vim radiosurgery for right-sided refractory tremor. (From Najdenovska E, Tuleasca C, Jorge J, et al. Comparison of MRI-based automated segmentation methods and functional neurosurgery targeting with direct visualization of the Ventro-intermediate thalamic nucleus at 7T. Sci Rep. 2019;9(1):1119; with permission.)

boundaries were overestimated and volumes were underestimated on 3 T compared with 7 T (**Fig. 29**). These findings could lead to inaccuracies in DBS and have significant ramifications, showing the value that 7 T can provide in a clinical setting.

LIMITATIONS

Although these advances with high-resolution 7 T show promise, there are also limitations that must be considered in clinical use. Artifacts seen with lower magnet strengths are exacerbated at 7 T, resulting in further image degradation.[59] For example, RF field inhomogeneities (B1) are significant at 7 T but less problematic at lower magnet strengths.[1] This difference can lead to both changes in contrast and decreased SNR.[74,89] B0 inhomogeneities, which increase

with increased field strength, are also a major limitation, leading to geometric distortions through susceptibility artifact. This limitation can be mitigated through shimming and decreased voxel volumes.[74] Another limitation is the design of the head coil, which, because of lack of a transmit body coil, has an increasingly complex design incorporating both transmit and receive elements.[74] In addition, at higher field strengths, there is an increase in the SAR, which exposes the patient to increased levels of heat.[74] In turn, this can cause patient discomfort and even RF-related burns.[97] Other limitations include artifact caused by chemical shift, which is detrimental to MRS, where the useable volume at 7 T is decreased.[74,89] In addition, compared with 3 T, there are different relaxation constants for T1W,

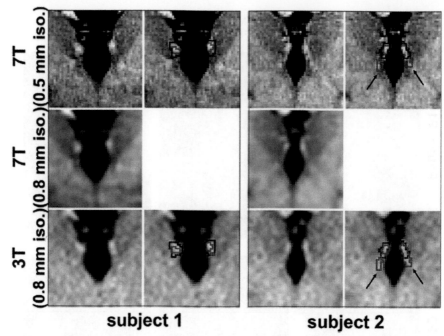

Fig. 29. Coronal coregistered 7-T MP2RAGE (*top*), downsampled 7-T MP2RAGE (*middle*), and 3-T T1W (*bottom*) imaging of the habenula with segmentation (blue and red outlines represent 7-T and 3-T segmentation, respectively). This comparison shows subtle overestimation on 3 T compared with 7 T. The black arrows show 3-T overestimation of the fascicula retroflexus. (*From* Kim JW, Naidich TP, Joseph J, et al. Reproducibility of myelin content-based human habenula segmentation at 3 Tesla. Hum Brain Mapp. 2018;39(7):3058–3071; with permission.)

T2W, and T2*-weighted imaging, which can affect both SNR and contrast.[74] In spite of these general limitations, 7 T can be used for lesion detection and anatomic visualization in both neurodegenerative and neuropsychiatric disease evaluation and management.

DISCLOSURES

V. Yedavalli, P. DiGiacomo, E. Tong: no disclosures. M. Zeineh received research funding from GE Healthcare.

REFERENCES

1. Kerchner GA. Ultra-high field 7T MRI: a new tool for studying Alzheimers disease. J Alzheimer's Dis 2011;26(SUPPL. 3):91–5.
2. Cosottini M, Frosini D, Pesaresi I, et al. Comparison of 3T and 7T susceptibility-weighted angiography of the substantia nigra in diagnosing Parkinson disease. Am J Neuroradiol 2015;36(3):461–6.
3. Wisse LEM, Gerritsen L, Zwanenburg JJM, et al. Subfields of the hippocampal formation at 7 T MRI: in vivo volumetric assessment. Neuroimage 2012; 61(4):1043–9.
4. Hammond KE, Metcalf M, Carvajal L, et al. Quantitative in vivo magnetic resonance imaging of multiple sclerosis at 7 Tesla with sensitivity to iron. Ann Neurol 2008;64(6):707–13.
5. Abosch A, Yacoub E, Ugurbil K, et al. An assessment of current brain targets for deep brain stimulation surgery with susceptibility-weighted imaging at 7 Tesla. Neurosurgery 2010;67(6):1745–56.
6. Goubran M, Rudko DA, Santyr B, et al. In vivo normative atlas of the hippocampal subfields using multi-echo susceptibility imaging at 7 Tesla. Hum Brain Mapp 2014;35(8):3588–601.
7. Bian W, Kerr AB, Tranvinh E, et al. MR susceptibility contrast imaging using a 2D simultaneous multi-slice gradient-echo sequence at 7T. PLoS One 2019;14(7):e0219705.
8. Liu T, Spincemaille P, De Rochefort L, et al. Calculation of susceptibility through multiple orientation sampling (COSMOS): a method for conditioning the inverse problem from measured magnetic field map to susceptibility source image in MRI. Magn Reson Med 2009;61(1):196–204.
9. Liu T, Liu J, De Rochefort L, et al. Morphology enabled dipole inversion (MEDI) from a single-angle acquisition: comparison with COSMOS in human brain imaging. Magn Reson Med 2011;66(3): 777–83.

10. Deistung A, Schäfer A, Schweser F, et al. Toward in vivo histology: a comparison of quantitative susceptibility mapping (QSM) with magnitude-, phase-, and R2*-imaging at ultra-high magnetic field strength. Neuroimage 2013;65:299–314.

11. Spincemaille P, Anderson J, Wu G, et al. Quantitative susceptibility mapping: MRI at 7T versus 3T. J Neuroimaging 2020;30(1):65–75.

12. Mattern H, Sciarra A, Lüsebrink F, et al. Prospective motion correction improves high-resolution quantitative susceptibility mapping at 7T. Magn Reson Med 2019;81(3):1605–19.

13. Di Ieva A, Göd S, Grabner G, et al. Three-dimensional susceptibility-weighted imaging at 7 T using fractal-based quantitative analysis to grade gliomas. Neuroradiology 2013;55(1):35–40.

14. Bian W, Tranvinh E, Tourdias T, et al. In vivo 7T MR quantitative susceptibility mapping reveals opposite susceptibility contrast between cortical and white matter lesions in multiple sclerosis. Am J Neuroradiol 2016;37(10):1808–15.

15. Zweckstetter M, Holak TA. An adiabatic multiple spin-echo pulse sequence: removal of systematic errors due to pulse imperfections and off-resonance effects. J Magn Reson 1998;133(1):134–47.

16. Emmerich J, Flassbeck S, Schmidt S, et al. Rapid and accurate dictionary-based T_2 mapping from multi-echo turbo spin echo data at 7 Tesla. J Magn Reson Imaging 2019;49(5):1253–62.

17. Maruyama S, Fukunaga M, Fautz HP, et al. Comparison of 3T and 7T MRI for the visualization of globus pallidus sub-segments. Sci Rep 2019;9(1):18357.

18. Zeineh MM, Parekh MB, Zaharchuk G, et al. Ultra-high-resolution imaging of the human brain with phase-cycled balanced steady-state free precession at 7 T. Invest Radiol 2014;49(5):278–89.

19. van Kalleveen IML, Koning W, Boer VO, et al. Adiabatic turbo spin echo in human applications at 7 T. Magn Reson Med 2012;68(2):580–7.

20. Polak D, Setsompop K, Cauley SF, et al. Wave-CAIPI for highly accelerated MP-RAGE imaging. Magn Reson Med 2018;79(1):401–6.

21. Seiger R, Hahn A, Hummer A, et al. Voxel-based morphometry at ultra-high fields. a comparison of 7T and 3T MRI data. Neuroimage 2015;113:207–16.

22. Marques JP, Kober T, Krueger G, et al. MP2RAGE, a self bias-field corrected sequence for improved segmentation and T1-mapping at high field. Neuroimage 2010;49(2):1271–81.

23. O'Brien KR, Kober T, Hagmann P, et al. Robust T1-weighted structural brain imaging and morphometry at 7T using MP2RAGE. PLoS One 2014;9(6):e99676.

24. Choi US, Kawaguchi H, Matsuoka Y, et al. Brain tissue segmentation based on MP2RAGE multi-contrast images in 7 T MRI. PLoS One 2019;14(2):e0210803.

25. Umutlu L, Theysohn N, Maderwald S, et al. 7 Tesla MPRAGE imaging of the intracranial arterial vasculature: nonenhanced versus contrast-enhanced. Acad Radiol 2013;20(5):628–34.

26. Tourdias T, Saranathan M, Levesque IR, et al. Visualization of intra-thalamic nuclei with optimized white-matter-nulled MPRAGE at 7T. Neuroimage 2014;84:534–45.

27. Planche V, Su JH, Mournet S, et al. White-matter-nulled MPRAGE at 7T reveals thalamic lesions and atrophy of specific thalamic nuclei in multiple sclerosis. Mult Scler 2020;26(8):987–92.

28. Lee J, Fukunaga M, Duyn JH. Improving contrast to noise ratio of resonance frequency contrast images (phase images) using balanced steady-state free precession. Neuroimage 2011;54(4):2779–88.

29. Bieri O, Scheffler K. On the origin of apparent low tissue signals in balanced SSFP. Magn Reson Med 2006;56(5):1067–74.

30. Elliott AM, Bernstein MA, Ward HA, et al. Nonlinear averaging reconstruction method for phase-cycle SSFP. Magn Reson Imaging 2007;25(3):359–64.

31. Ribot EJ, Wecker D, Trotier AJ, et al. Water selective imaging and bSSFP banding artifact correction in humans and small animals at 3T and 7T, respectively. PLoS One 2015;10(10):e0139249.

32. Parekh MB, Rutt BK, Purcell R, et al. Ultra-high resolution in-vivo 7.0T structural imaging of the human hippocampus reveals the endfolial pathway. Neuroimage 2015;112:1–6.

33. Gallichan D, Marques JP, Gruetter R. Retrospective correction of involuntary microscopic head movement using highly accelerated fat image navigators (3D FatNavs) at 7T. Magn Reson Med 2016;75(3):1030–9.

34. Engström M, Mårtensson M, Avventi E, et al. Collapsed fat navigators for brain 3D rigid body motion. Magn Reson Imaging 2015;33(8):984–91.

35. Gallichan D, Marques JP. Optimizing the acceleration and resolution of three-dimensional fat image navigators for high-resolution motion correction at 7T. Magn Reson Med 2017;77(2):547–58.

36. Federau C, Gallichan D. Motion-correction enabled ultra-high resolution in-vivo 7T-MRI of the brain. PLoS One 2016;11(5):e0154974.

37. Ooi MB, Krueger S, Thomas WJ, et al. Prospective real-time correction for arbitrary head motion using active markers. Magn Reson Med 2009;62(4):943–54.

38. Vannesjo SJ, Wilm BJ, Duerst Y, et al. Retrospective correction of physiological field fluctuations in high-field brain MRI using concurrent field monitoring. Magn Reson Med 2015;73(5):1833–43.

39. Haeberlin M, Kasper L, Barmet C, et al. Real-time motion correction using gradient tones and head-mounted NMR field probes. Magn Reson Med 2015;74(3):647–60.

40. White N, Roddey C, Shankaranarayanan A, et al. PROMO: real-time prospective motion correction in MRI using image-based tracking. Magn Reson Med 2010;63(1):91–105.

41. Schulz J, Siegert T, Reimer E, et al. An embedded optical tracking system for motion-corrected magnetic resonance imaging at 7T. Magn Reson Mater Physics Biol Med 2012;25(6):443–53.

42. Maclaren J, Armstrong BSR, Barrows RT, et al. Measurement and correction of microscopic head motion during magnetic resonance imaging of the brain. PLoS One 2012;7(11):e48088.

43. Zaitsev M, Dold C, Sakas G, et al. Magnetic resonance imaging of freely moving objects: prospective real-time motion correction using an external optical motion tracking system. Neuroimage 2006;31(3):1038–50.

44. Speck O, Hennig J, Zaitsev M. Prospective real-time slice-by-slice motion correction for fMRI in freely moving subjects. MAGMA 2006;19(2):55–61. https://doi.org/10.1007/s10334-006-0027-1.

45. Maclaren J, Aksoy M, Ooi MB, et al. Prospective motion correction using coil-mounted cameras: cross-calibration considerations. Magn Reson Med 2018;79(4):1911–21.

46. Spangler-Bickell MG, Zeineh M, Jansen F, et al. Rigid motion correction for brain PET/MR imaging using optical tracking. IEEE Trans Radiat Plasma Med Sci 2018;3(4):498–503.

47. Stucht D, Danishad KA, Schulze P, et al. Highest resolution in vivo human brain MRI using prospective motion correction. PLoS One 2015;10(7):e0133921.

48. Mattern H, Sciarra A, Godenschweger F, et al. Prospective motion correction enables highest resolution time-of-flight angiography at 7T. Magn Reson Med 2018;80(1):248–58.

49. Morel A, Magnin M, Jeanmonod D. Multiarchitectonic and stereotactic atlas of the human thalamus. J Comp Neurol 1997;387(4):588–630.

50. DiGiacomo P, Maclaren J, Aksoy M, et al. A within-coil optical prospective motion-correction system for brain imaging at 7T. Magn Reson Med 2020;84(3):1661–71.

51. Mori S, Aggarwal M. In vivo magnetic resonance imaging of the human limbic white matter. Front Aging Neurosci 2014;6:321.

52. Derix J, Yang S, Lüsebrink F, et al. Visualization of the amygdalo-hippocampal border and its structural variability by 7T and 3T magnetic resonance imaging. Hum Brain Mapp 2014;35(9):4316–29.

53. Thomas BP, Welch EB, Niederhauser BD, et al. High-resolution 7T MRI of the human hippocampus in vivo. J Magn Reson Imaging 2008;28(5):1266–72.

54. Ding SL, Van Hoesen GW. Organization and detailed parcellation of human hippocampal head and body regions based on a combined analysis of Cyto- and chemoarchitecture. J Comp Neurol 2015;523(15):2233–53.

55. Zeineh MM, Palomero-Gallagher N, Axer M, et al. Direct visualization and mapping of the spatial course of fiber tracts at microscopic resolution in the human hippocampus. Cereb Cortex 2017;27(3):1779–94.

56. Wisse LEM, Kuijf HJ, Honingh AM, et al. Automated hippocampal subfield segmentation at 7T MRI. Am J Neuroradiol 2016;37(6):1050–7.

57. Sladky R, Baldinger P, Kranz GS, et al. High-resolution functional MRI of the human amygdala at 7 T. Eur J Radiol 2013;82(5):728–33.

58. Cavedo E, Boccardi M, Ganzola R, et al. Local amygdala structural differences with 3T MRI in patients with Alzheimer disease. Neurology 2011;76(8):727–33.

59. McKiernan EF, O'Brien JT. 7T MRI for neurodegenerative dementias in vivo: a systematic review of the literature. J Neurol Neurosurg Psychiatry 2017;88(7):564–74.

60. Ali R, Goubran M, Choudhri O, et al. Seven-Tesla MRI and neuroimaging biomarkers for Alzheimer's disease. Neurosurg Focus 2015;39(5):E4.

61. Kerchner GA, Hess CP, Hammond-Rosenbluth KE, et al. Hippocampal CA1 apical neuropil atrophy in mild Alzheimer disease visualized with 7-T MRI. Neurology 2010;75(15):1381–7.

62. Kerchner GA, Deutsch GK, Zeineh M, et al. Hippocampal CA1 apical neuropil atrophy and memory performance in Alzheimer's disease. Neuroimage 2012;63(1):194–202.

63. Kerchner GA, Berdnik D, Shen JC, et al. APOE e4 worsens hippocampal CA1 apical neuropil atrophy and episodic memory. Neurology 2014;82(8):691–7.

64. Khan UA, Liu L, Provenzano FA, et al. Molecular drivers and cortical spread of lateral entorhinal cortex dysfunction in preclinical Alzheimer's disease. Nat Neurosci 2014;17(2):304–11.

65. Wisse LEM, Reijmer YD, Ter Telgte A, et al. Hippocampal disconnection in early Alzheimer's disease: a 7 tesla MRI study. J Alzheimer's Dis 2015;45(4):1247–56.

66. Boutet C, Chupin M, Lehéricy S, et al. Detection of volume loss in hippocampal layers in Alzheimer's disease using 7 T MRI: a feasibility study. Neuroimage Clin 2014;5:341–8.

67. van Rooden S, Versluis MJ, Liem MK, et al. Cortical phase changes in Alzheimer's disease at 7T MRI: a novel imaging marker. Alzheimer's Dement 2014;10(1):e19–26.

68. Zeineh MM, Chen Y, Kitzler HH, et al. Activated iron-containing microglia in the human hippocampus identified by magnetic resonance imaging in Alzheimer disease. Neurobiol Aging 2015;36(9):2483–500.

69. Kenkhuis B, Jonkman LE, Bulk M, et al. 7T MRI allows detection of disturbed cortical lamination of

the medial temporal lobe in patients with Alzheimer's disease. Neuroimage Clin 2019;21:101665.

70. Colon AJ, va Osch MJP, Buijs M, et al. MEG-guided analysis of 7T-MRI in patients with epilepsy. Seizure 2018;60:29–38.

71. Breyer T, Wanke I, Maderwald S, et al. Imaging of patients with hippocampal sclerosis at 7 Tesla. Initial results. Acad Radiol 2010;17(4):421–6.

72. Griffiths PD, Coley SC, Connolly DJA, et al. MR imaging of patients with localisation-related seizures: initial experience at 3.0T and relevance to the NICE guidelines. Clin Radiol 2005;60(10):1090–9.

73. Feldman RE, Delman BN, Pawha PS, et al. 7T MRI in epilepsy patients with previously normal clinical MRI exams compared against healthy controls. PLoS One 2019;14(3):e0213642.

74. Balchandani P, Naidich TP. Ultra-high-field MR neuroimaging. Am J Neuroradiol 2015;36(7):1204–15.

75. Knake S, Triantafyllou C, Wald LL, et al. 3T phased array MRI improves the presurgical evaluation in focal epilepsies: a prospective study. Neurology 2005;65(7):1026–31.

76. De Ciantis A, Barba C, Tassi L, et al. 7T MRI in focal epilepsy with unrevealing conventional field strength imaging. Epilepsia 2016;57(3):445–54.

77. Rutland JW, Feldman RE, Delman BN, et al. Subfield-specific tractography of the hippocampus in epilepsy patients at 7 Tesla. Seizure 2018;62:3–10.

78. Feldman RE, Rutland JW, Fields MC, et al. Quantification of perivascular spaces at 7 T: a potential MRI biomarker for epilepsy. Seizure 2018;54:11–8.

79. Springer E, Dymerska B, Cardoso PL, et al. Comparison of routine brain imaging at 3 T and 7 T. Invest Radiol 2016;51(8):469–82.

80. Stefanits H, Springer E, Pataraia E, et al. Seven-Tesla MRI of hippocampal sclerosis: an in vivo feasibility study with histological correlations. Invest Radiol 2017;52(11):666–71.

81. Gillmann C, Coras R, Rössler K, et al. Ultra-high field MRI of human hippocampi: morphological and multiparametric differentiation of hippocampal sclerosis subtypes. PLoS One 2018;13(4):e0196008.

82. Voets NL, Hodgetts CJ, Sen A, et al. Hippocampal MRS and subfield volumetry at 7T detects dysfunction not specific to seizure focus. Sci Rep 2017;7(1):1–14.

83. Eapen M, Zald DH, Gatenby JC, et al. Using high-resolution MR imaging at 7T to evaluate the anatomy of the midbrain dopaminergic system. Am J Neuroradiol 2011;32(4):688–94.

84. Blazejewska AI, Schwarz ST, Pitiot A, et al. Visualization of nigrosome 1 and its loss in PD: pathoanatomical correlation and in vivo 7 T MRI. Neurology 2013;81(6):534–40.

85. Cosottini M, Frosini D, Pesaresi I, et al. MR imaging of the substantia nigra at 7 T enables diagnosis of parkinson disease. Radiology 2014;271(3):831–8.

86. Poston KL, Ua Cruadhlaoich MAI, Santoso LF, et al. Substantia nigra volume dissociates bradykinesia and rigidity from tremor in Parkinson's disease: A 7 Tesla Imaging Study. J Parkinsons Dis 2020;10(2):591–604.

87. Brown SSG, Rutland JW, Verma G, et al. Structural MRI at 7T reveals amygdala nuclei and hippocampal subfield volumetric association with major depressive disorder symptom severity. Sci Rep 2019;9(1):1–10.

88. Johnston BA, Steele JD, Tolomeo S, et al. Structural MRI-based predictions in patients with treatment-refractory depression (TRD). PLoS One 2015;10(7):e0132958.

89. Morris LS, Kundu P, Costi S, et al. Ultra-high field MRI reveals mood-related circuit disturbances in depression: a comparison between 3-Tesla and 7-Tesla. Transl Psychiatry 2019;9(1):94.

90. Liu Y, D'Haese PF, Newton AT, et al. Generation of human thalamus atlases from 7 T data and application to intrathalamic nuclei segmentation in clinical 3 T T1-weighted images. Magn Reson Imaging 2020;65:114–28.

91. Kanowski M, Voges J, Buentjen L, et al. Direct visualization of anatomic subfields within the superior aspect of the human lateral thalamus by MRI at 7T. Am J Neuroradiol 2014;35(9):1721–7.

92. Najdenovska E, Tuleasca C, Jorge J, et al. Comparison of MRI-based automated segmentation methods and functional neurosurgery targeting with direct visualization of the ventro-intermediate thalamic nucleus at 7T. Sci Rep 2019;9(1):1119.

93. Lenglet C, Abosch A, Yacoub E, et al. Comprehensive in vivo mapping of the human basal ganglia and thalamic connectome in individuals using 7T MRI. PLoS One 2012;7(1):e29153.

94. Xiao YZ, Zitella LM, Duchin Y, et al. Multimodal 7T imaging of thalamic nuclei for preclinical deep brain stimulation applications. Front Neurosci 2016;10:264.

95. Strotmann B, Heidemann RM, Anwander A, et al. High-resolution MRI and diffusion-weighted imaging of the human habenula at 7 Tesla. J Magn Reson Imaging 2014;39(4):1018–26.

96. Kim JW, Naidich TP, Joseph J, et al. Reproducibility of myelin content-based human habenula segmentation at 3 Tesla. Hum Brain Mapp 2018;39(7):3058–71.

97. Allison J, Yanasak N. What MRI sequences produce the highest specific absorption rate (SAR), and is there something we should be doing to reduce the SAR during standard examinations? Am J Roentgenol 2015;205(2):W140.

UltraHigh Field MR Imaging in Epilepsy

Gaurav Verma, PhD[a],*, Bradley N. Delman, MD, MS[b], Priti Balchandani, PhD[a,b]

KEYWORDS

- 7T • Epilepsy • Ultrahigh • MR imaging

KEY POINTS

- MR imaging at ultrahigh field strengths, often defined as 7T or greater, has gained increasing interest in clinical imaging.
- Among the most promising clinical applications of ultrahigh field imaging is the characterization and treatment planning of epilepsy.
- Minimally invasive alternatives to surgery have also emerged, including responsive neuromodulation and deep brain stimulation.

INTRODUCTION

MR imaging at ultrahigh field strengths, often defined as 7T or greater, has gained increasing interest in clinical imaging, particularly following the first 510(k) approval of a 7T MR imaging scanner by the Food and Drug Administration in 2017 (Terra 7T, Siemens Healthineers, Erlangen, Germany). As of June 2020, at least 88 in vivo human MR imaging scanners of 7T or greater have been installed worldwide, including both research and clinical units. Higher field strengths facilitate proportional gains in signal-to-noise ratio (SNR) over lower field strengths,[1,2] which in turn may be leveraged for higher imaging resolution, greater tissue contrast or faster scan times, or some combination thereof. These gains may confer improved sensitivity in various advanced imaging applications to improve detection or characterization of small or poorly differentiated imaging features.[3,4]

Among the most promising clinical applications of ultrahigh field imaging is the characterization and treatment planning of epilepsy. Affecting up to 1% of the total population, epilepsy is a heterogeneous group of neurologic disorders associated with recurrent seizures.[5] There is also mounting evidence that epilepsy is a complex network disease with long-term frequent seizures causing changes in the brain beyond the primary epileptic regions into other areas affected by seizure activity.[6–9] Factors such as seizure frequency, severity and duration of disease, and seizure severity all contribute to the breadth of abnormalities that underlie these seizure networks.[8,10–17]

In the one-third of patients in whom antiepilepsy drugs are ineffective, ablative or resective surgery may be considered. Minimally invasive alternatives to surgery have also emerged, including responsive neuromodulation (RNS) and deep brain stimulation. The success of these targeted interventions critically depends on the localization of seizure onset zones (SOZs), typically through neuroimaging. Although several epilepsy cases exhibit focal lesions at conventional field strengths, in about one-third of patients with refractory epilepsy lesions are not identified on routine clinical imaging.[18] Identifying the SOZs in these patients may require more advanced techniques to detect smaller or more subtle imaging features. These subtle imaging findings may include cortical abnormalities (including migrational disorders), atrophy, or asymmetry in subcortical structures.[19] Although not suspected to cause seizure activity, abnormally large or numerous perivascular spaces

[a] Biomedical Engineering and Imaging Institute, The Icahn School of Medicine at Mount Sinai, 1470 Madison Avenue, New York, NY 10029, USA; [b] Department of Diagnostic, Molecular and Interventional Radiology, The Icahn School of Medicine at Mount Sinai, One Gustave L. Levy Place, Box 1234, New York, NY 10029, USA
* Corresponding author.
E-mail address: gaurav.verma@mssm.edu

Magn Reson Imaging Clin N Am 29 (2021) 41–52
https://doi.org/10.1016/j.mric.2020.09.006

(PVS) may also be a biomarker for epilepsy, whichindicates regional volume loss[20] or inflammatory activity.[21]

Advanced MR imaging techniques such as susceptibility weighted imaging (SWI), diffusion-weighted (DWI) or diffusion tensor imaging (DTI), and functional MR (fMR) imaging each benefit from the SNR advantages at ultrahigh field.[22] SWI also receives the further benefit of higher susceptibility at ultrahigh field to improve lesional conspicuity. DTI, DWI, and fMR imaging heavily depend on gradient performance, and newer ultrahigh field scanners typically use more powerful gradients for the benefit of these techniques. These advanced imaging techniques at ultrahigh field may facilitate improved subtyping of epilepsy through the detection vascular abnormalities or irregularities in structural or functional connectivity.[23,24]

IMAGING MODALITIES

High-resolution structural and functional sequences are required to analyze subregions of the hippocampus, amygdala, and thalamus, which may act as sensitive markers for seizure pathology and more accurate targets for deep brain stimulation (DBS) and RNS therapies.[25–30] The addition of high-resolution functional and structural connectivity analysis with fMR imaging and DWI/DTI, respectively, has been shown to clarify regions of the brain involved in abnormal seizure activity when analyzed alongside structural images.[7,23,31–36] Magnetic resonance spectroscopic imaging (MRSI) captures signal from metabolites such as N-acetyl aspartate (NAA) and creatine (Cr) to provide information about neuronal integrity and total energy metabolism. MRSI studies have shown that NAA levels may be used to lateralize and localize the brain regions where the seizures originate in temporal lobe epilepsy (TLE).[37–39] Ultrahigh field MR imaging significantly increases the sensitivity of all of these neuroimaging modalities and enables image acquisitions at appreciably finer resolution.[22] **Table 1** summarizes the value of each of these methods at 7T for epilepsy. Multimodal preoperative MR imaging at 7T should also result in improved placement of intracranial electroencephalogram (iEEG). Stereo-EEG (SEEG) is a technique that allows for collection of iEEG data from virtually any location in the brain with great precision and could benefit significantly from high-resolution multimodal imaging. Improved diagnostic accuracy of such an implant may lead to greater success in the following resective surgery, ablative surgery, or neuromodulation treatment of the epileptic network. This results in decreased infection rates and increased monitoring accuracy, reducing the duration of hospital stays.[40–42]

Structural Imaging

The most basic applications of MR imaging uses inherent differences in tissue T_1 and T_2 relaxation properties to generate image contrast. Examples include magnetization-prepared rapid gradient echo (MPRAGE) based on T1-weighting and fast spin echo or turbo spin echo (TSE) based on T_2-weighting. A variant of T2-weighting called fluid-attenuated inversion recovery (FLAIR) uses an inversion pulse to lower the signal of normal cerebrospinal fluid (CSF) to increase conspicuity of edema especially near bulk fluid. Reviews of published ultrahigh field research generally reveal improved resolution compared with lower field strengths, with T1-weighted imaging yielding submillimeter isotropic resolution and 2-dimensional (2D) T2-weighted imaging also producing in-plane resolution well under 1 mm. Clinically, ultrahigh field imaging has demonstrated improved visualization of subtle features such as malformations of cortical development[43] compared with lower field strengths. Still other novel structural imaging contrasts have been developed including fast gray matter acquisition T1 inversion recovery (FGATIR), which improves gray matter-white matter contrast through selective suppression of white matter signal with inversion recovery pulses.[44]

Although T2 TSE and T2 FLAIR can potentially offer higher SNR than lower field strengths, techniques must also recognize and accommodate the associated increase specific absorption rate (SAR) that high field imaging imparts (see section 4.2). SAR limitations can, therefore, temper some of the putative ultrahigh field gains. **Fig. 1** shows hippocampal subfields of a 27-year-old female patient with MTLE segmented with the benefit of higher resolution at 7T. The patient was both qualitatively observed to have asymmetric hippocampus on clinical assessment and showed increased asymmetry on quantitative anatomic segmentation.

Susceptibility Weighted Imaging

SWI and the related quantitative susceptibility mapping take advantage of the susceptibility differences caused by the paramagnetic, diamagnetic, and ferromagnetic properties of local tissues. As magnetic susceptibility increases proportionately with field strength, SWI benefits greatly from ultrahigh fields. SWI uses the paramagnetic properties of deoxygenated blood to visualize tissue vasculature, reducing signal in

Technique	Advantage at 7T	Abnormalities Detected and Imaging Markers
T1	Increased SNR enables higher isotropic resolution	Cortical, migrational, and hippocampal abnormalities. Hippocampal subfield and thalamic subnuclei volumetrics
T2	Increased SNR and enhanced contrast results in increased conspicuity of lesions	Cortical abnormalities (dysplasias, malformations, heterotopias), hippocampal sclerosis, lesions. Hippocampal subfield and thalamic subnuclei volumetrics
SWI	Increased sensitivity to susceptibility effects and venous anomalies	Vascular lesions, hypervascularity, and cavernomas, associated with or acting as seizure source
MRSI	Increased SNR and spectral separation	Neuronal loss detected through NAA/Cr levels
dMR imaging	Increased SNR. Hippocampal subfield-specific connectivity may be performed	Abnormal structural connectivity underlying seizure networks Hippocampal subfield-specific tract density
fMR imaging	Increased SNR and BOLD contrast	Abnormal functional connectivity in seizure networks

Table 1
MR imaging modality, advantage at 7T, and detected epileptogenic abnormalities

postcapillary vessels so they appear darker than surrounding tissues. SWI is also useful for detection of microhemorrhages and of vascular, iron-rich, or calcified lesions such as cavernous malformations.[45] One study exploiting SWI in drug-resistant lesional epilepsy patients[46] demonstrated the ability of SWI to identify focal thickening and abnormal vasculature such as tortuous veins, which may be implicated in the pathogenesis of epilepsy. A second study identified abnormal blood vessel morphology and reduced gray-white contrast and presence of thin vessels in the regions of tuberous sclerosis.[47]

Diffusion-Weighted Imaging and Diffusion Tensor Imaging

Diffusion-based imaging techniques, including DWI and DTI, probe the structural connectivity of brain tissue by characterizing diffusion restriction of water molecules in the presence of an applied directional magnetic gradient. DWI and DTI receive a nominal SNR benefit of ultrahigh field, so these gradient-dependent techniques separately benefit from the better gradient performance typical in these newer MR imaging systems. Because of its greater directional specificity, DTI can be used for fiber tractography through sophisticated reconstruction algorithms, such as those

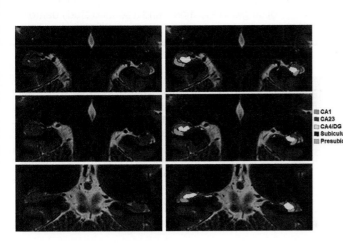

Fig. 1. Hippocampal subfield segmentation of a patient with MTLE overlayed on coronal-oblique T2-weighted TSE image acquired at 7T. At left are 3 unmarked slices of TSE images. At right are segmented cornu ammonis 1 (CA1), cornu ammonis 2 + 3 (CA2/3), cornu ammonis 4 + dentate gyrus (CA4/DG), subiculum, and presubiculum.

offered by MRtrix3 (Brain Research Institute, Melbourne, VIC, Australia). These techniques can leverage constrained spherical deconvolution to calculate fiber orientation distributions and resolve crossing fibers. From preselected volumetric seeds, for example, within individual hippocampal subfields,[25] tractography can elucidate the structural connectivity between the hippocampal subfields and other parts of the brain. With adequate resolution afforded by the high-performance magnetic gradients, a strong main field at ultrahigh field strengths, DTI tractography, can potentially identify epileptogenic foci in patients whose seizure onset zones are otherwise poorly visualized through conventional imaging.[48,49] **Fig. 2** shows whole-brain tractography performed using TractSeg (German Cancer Research Center, Heidelberg, Germany) and displayed using MrTrix3 with 7T DTI data acquired from a patient with TLE. Red, green, and blue coloring is incorporated reflecting predominantly left-right, anterior-posterior, and superior-inferior fiber directionality, respectively. **Figs. 3 and 4** show reconstructed seeded tractography performed by MRTrix3 superimposed against a coregistered structural T1-weighted MR imaging. **Fig. 3** shows cortical, limbic, and corticolimbic tractography, whereas **Fig. 4** shows tractography specific to segmented hippocampal subfields. Fiber coloring follows a typical MR convention, where fiber orientation is encoded as red, green, and blue to reflect left-right, anterior-posterior, and superior-inferior fibers, respectively.

Functional MR Imaging

fMR imaging uses a time designated series of images to measure the blood oxygenation level–dependent (BOLD) response. Task-dependent BOLD imaging characterizes changes in blood flow and oxygenation elucidated by alternating task and rest periods to determine changes in relative vascular oxygenation, with vascular susceptibility varying between paramagnetic deoxygenated blood and diamagnetic oxygenated

blood. Of increasing interest is resting state fMR imaging, in which low-frequency cycling can be leveraged to characterize functional connectivity among brain regions.[50,51] Ultrahigh field imaging may improve on lower field techniques because fMR imaging enjoys better than linear gains in susceptibility in proportion to field strength. One comparison study between 3T and 7T demonstrated up to 3 times improvements in SNR and resting-state functional connectivity coefficients at the higher field.[52] Another study of patients with mesial TLE (MTLE) using BOLD fMR imaging at 7T[53] demonstrated functional network asymmetry among patients with TLE in the region around the mesial temporal lobe.

Magnetic Resonance Spectroscopic Imaging

MRSI assays the metabolic composition of tissue by detecting subtle differences in resonance frequency according to the molecular environment around atomic nuclei. These differences, called chemical shifts, stem from partial shielding or deshielding of the observed magnetic field due to the electrons in the surrounding molecular structure. MRSI receives a double benefit from ultrahigh field, with proportional gains in both SNR and spectral separation, facilitating better differentiation and quantification of metabolite signals.[54–56] Because spatial localization of a volume of interest is typically performed using 180° refocusing radiofrequency (RF) pulses in MRSI, the technique is highly sensitive to B_1 inhomogeneity, leading to the implementation of B_1-insensitive semiadiabatic techniques[57] to compensate.

Studies using MRSI at 7T in patients with epilepsy have demonstrated that metabolic abnormalities may be present in the epileptogenic region.[58–61] For example, one study demonstrated improved surgical outcomes in patients in whom metabolic abnormality was detected in the region of surgical resection[59] and a second study demonstrated abnormalities in the ratio between NAA and Cr among patients withMTLE.[58]

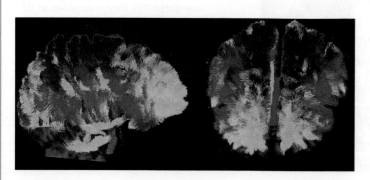

Fig. 2. Sagittal (left) and coronal-oblique (right) images showing whole-brain tractography performed using TractSeg and displayed with MRTrix3 using 7T DTI data from a patient with epilepsy. Red, green, and blue coloring represents fibers whose dominant orientations are left-right, anterior-posterior, and superior-inferior, respectively.

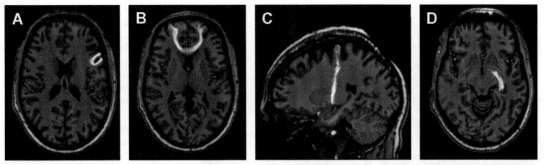

Fig. 3. Seed-based tractography images from DTI scan of patient with epilepsy at 7T. Shown are U-fiber bundle between adjacent cortical nodes (*A*), long-range fibers connecting distant cortical nodes (*B*), corticolimbic tract (*C*), and interlimbic tract (*D*).

IMAGING FEATURES
Focal Cortical Dysplasia

Focal cortical dysplasia (FCD) is a congenital abnormality that may be manifested clinically as drug-resistant epilepsy and a common target for resective surgery in these patients. A 7T study of patients suspected of FCD[62] demonstrated the superiority of ultrahigh field imaging in detecting these lesions. Structural 7T MR imaging identified all the lesions previously seen at 1.5T and 3T, yet also detected additional lesions undetected at those lower fields. That study suggested T2 FLAIR showed the best visualization of FCD lesions among the commonly applied structural MR imaging contrasts. **Fig. 5** coronal oblique T2-

weighted TSE and axial SWI images showing focal cortical defect in 19-year-old male patient with epilepsy.

Hippocampal Sclerosis

Hippocampal sclerosis is the prototypical pathology in MTLE, in reports from surgery and autopsy. Hippocampal sclerosis appears on structural imaging as diminished volume (atrophy) within the whole hippocampus or its component subfields, as well as a disruption in the laminar architecture with associated signal changes. Automated segmentation algorithms, such as FreeSurfer[63] and automated segmentation of hippocampal subfields,[64] have been developed in recent years to

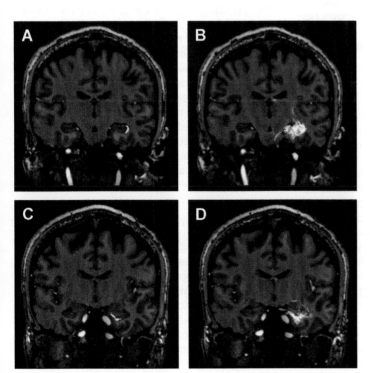

Fig. 4. Hippocampal subfield-specific tractography overlayed on T1-weighted MPRAGE imaging and generated using 7T DTI data acquired from a patient with epilepsy. Shown are coronal slice with CA1 overlay in yellow (*A*) and subiculum overlay (*C*). Seeded tractography from CA1 and subiculum are shown in *B* and *D*, respectively.

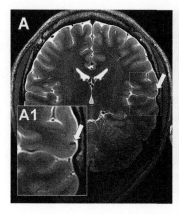
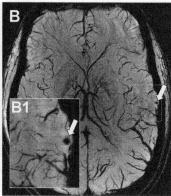

Fig. 5. Focal cortical defect in a 19-year-old man with history of generalized tonic-clonic convulsions (GTCC). Coronal T2 TSE-weighted image demonstrates a 3-mm hypervascular cortical malformation in the left frontal operculum, manifested as an area of diminished signal (*arrows* in A and in the magnified inset A1, whose location is indicated by dashed box in A). This area blooms to a larger size and conspicuity on a minimum intensity projection of susceptibility weighted imaging (*arrows* in B and in the magnified inset B1, using the same localizing conventions).

quantify the volume of the hippocampi and their subfields, using a probabilistic approach based on voxel position and contrast. A tissue-contrast–based segmentation approach would likely benefit from the improved contrast offered by ultrahigh field imaging, and multiple studies have consequently reported reliable segmentation of hippocampal subfields at 7T.[25,61,65,66]

Studies of hippocampal sclerosis at 7T[67–70] demonstrated correlation between MTLE and ipsilateral sclerosis of the hippocampus with manual segmentation.[69] These studies also revealed some limitations of ultrahigh field scanners in imaging the hippocampus including increased field B_1 field inhomogeneity in the region and limitations on minimum repetition time for high RF power sequences due to the SAR limits. **Fig. 6** shows hippocampal asymmetry detected in a coronal-oblique T1-weighted MP2RAGE image acquired at 7T.

Polymicrogyria

Polymicrogyria (PMG) is a cortical malformation characterized by abnormally prominent infolding or nodularity of one or more cortical locations, giving rise to paradoxic thickening of the cortical band on imaging with fusion of the molecular layer across sulci. Although its pathogenesis is not well understood, causal factors include congenital infections, in utero ischemia and genetic mutations. PMG may be unilateral or bilateral, focal or diffuse, and symmetric or asymmetric and may be associated with epilepsy. Zones of PMG also serve as potential targets for surgical treatment of epilepsy. A study of 10 patients with polymicrogyria already diagnosed at 3T demonstrated improved visualization at 7T,[71] with SWI angiography revealing dilated superficial veins in association with the polymicrogyria. **Fig. 7** shows images of polymicrogyria acquired with multiple imaging modalities at 7T.

Perivascular Spaces

PVS are small fluid-filled spaces within white matter, which appear isointense to static CSF-filled regions on structural imaging. These spaces coincide with arterial trajectories, and excess size, number, or asymmetry may be a marker for neurologic disorders such as epilepsy. This prominence is attributed to regional volume loss. Because many are small or at least start small (perhaps a half-millimeter in transverse diameter or less) these spaces are more readily detected using high-resolution ultrahigh field imaging. In particular, 2D T_2 TSE, which shows high contrast between the CSF-filled spaces and the dark surrounding white matter, has been very effective in demonstrating regional variability in PVS. Manual segmentation of PVS revealed significant differences between the asymmetry index of PVS compared with healthy controls.[20] Because a single subject may exhibit hundreds or thousands of MR-visible PVS, particularly at ultrahigh field, segmentation of these spaces is a laborious process when performed manually and may benefit from automation based on imaging contrast. **Fig. 8** shows a zoomed in section of an axial T2-weighted TSE image showing the presence of multiple perivascular spaces, detected and marked by a manual reader.

TECHNICAL LIMITATIONS
B_1 Field Inhomogeneity

Ultrahigh field imaging suffers from poorer homogeneity of the applied B_1 RF field compared with lower field strengths. Image homogeneity results from the interaction between the radiofrequency pulses and the dielectric properties of the scanned tissue, including conductivity and permittivity. The shorter wavelengths at ultrahigh field can result in standing wave patterns of high and low

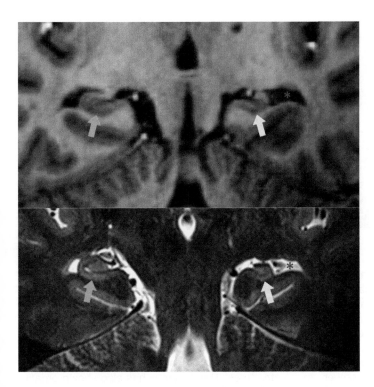

Fig. 6. Coronal-oblique T1-weighted MP2RAGE image (top) acquired at 7T with 0.7 mm³ isotropic resolution and T2-weighted TSE (bottom) with 0.4 mm in-plane resolution showing hippocampal asymmetry in a 64-year-old patient with intractable temporal lobe epilepsy. Both images show reduced left hippocampal volume (*yellow arrows*) compared with the normal configuration on the right (*blue arrows*). Larger than normal left temporal horn that indicates volume loss is marked by red asterisk.

interference within the scanned field of view, producing characteristic bright and dark regions in the image. The resultant inhomogeneity can be particularly problematic in the visualization of

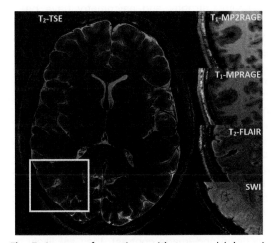

Fig. 7. Images of a patient with temporal lobe epilepsy showing polymicrogyria at 7T. The large image at left is an axial T2-weighted TSE image with 0.4 mm in-plane resolution and 2 mm slice thickness. The 4 images at right are T1-weighted MP2RAGE and MPRAGE (coronal-oblique, both with 0.7 mm isotropic resolution) along with axial T2-weighted FLAIR (0.4 mm in-plane resolution) and SWI (0.2 mm in-plane resolution).

deep brain structures and temporal lobe, complicating ultrahigh field imaging–based assessment of epilepsy. Multiple techniques have emerged for mitigating the effects of this inhomogeneity including B_1 insensitive adiabatic pulses[72–74] and parallel transmit (PTx) coils, which use multiple transmission elements working independently and predetermined B_1 field maps to compensate for inhomogeneity with hardware.[75] The use of high permittivity dielectric pads, such as a deuterium-based suspension of barium titanate,[76,77] have demonstrated improved coverage in regions with poor B_1-homogeneity at ultrahigh field strengths.

Specific Absorption Rate

RF power deposition scales with the square of the main field strength, making sequences using multiple 180-degree RF pulses such as T2 TSE and T2 FLAIR particularly SAR-intensive at ultrahigh fields. For these sequences, modification of technique to comply with Food and Drug Administration–designated guidelines for SAR (3.2 W/kg over 10 minutes for brain imaging) can impose restrictions on potential signal gains, which can then adversely affect resolution and scan time. SAR limitations further complicate strategies for mitigating B_1 inhomogeneity, because adiabatic pulses tend to be SAR intensive and

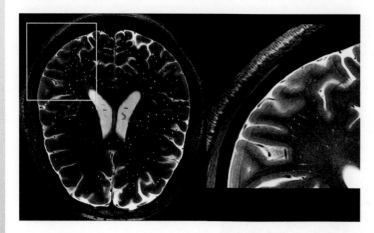

Fig. 8. Whole-brain axial T2-weighted TSE image (acquired at 7T with 0.4 mm in-plane resolution, 2.0 mm slice thickness) and zoomed-in section indicated by yellow square. Manually demarcated cross-sections of detected perivascular spaces are marked by yellow lines.

PTx coils[78] require complex calculations—and often restrictive approximations—to calculate the maximum local SAR. Although issues related to SAR are a major consideration across most applications of ultrahigh field imaging, they may be particularly limiting in epilepsy imaging due to the need to visualize deep brain structures, which typically require high transmission power to compensate for the poorer penetration of short-wavelength RF in the brain at ultrahigh field.

Other Limitations

To date, no commercial human 7T MR imaging system includes a body transmit RF coil, necessitating the integration of RF transmit elements into detection coils. These coils may thus exhibit RF localization effects with reduced sensitivity away from the coil elements—for example, in the skull base or brain stem region on birdcage head coils.

Anatomic imaging contrast depends on the T1 and T2 properties of the local tissue, which in turn depends on the B_0 field strength, and may not perfectly match the contrast of 1.5T and 3T clinical imaging systems. Adoption of ultrahigh field imaging for routine clinical imaging will require familiarization of clinicians to those contrasts, and automatic segmentation algorithms that depend on these contrasts may require specific calibration for ultrahigh field.

TECHNICAL ADVANCES
Deep Brain Stimulation

In recent years, DBS has received increasing clinical interest in the characterization and treatment of movement disorders and depression and has also demonstrated efficacy in reducing or eliminating seizures in refractory TLE without the need for surgical resection.[79–81] DBS treatment of epilepsy typically targets the thalamus and in

particular the anterior or centromedian subthalamic nuclei. Resolving these subthalamic structures is complicated by poor anatomic contrast on conventional imaging, yet may benefit from both the improved contrast at ultrahigh field and the implementation of high-contrast FGATIR[44] to improve visualization of these deep gray matter structures. The thalamus has also shown organization by fiber connectivity, and it may therefore be amenable to segmentation through clustering of DTI data including fiber direction or long distance connectivity.[82–86]

Advanced Postprocessing and Automated Segmentation

Volumetric atrophy and asymmetry have been implicated in several neurologic disorders including epilepsy.[53] This has led to increasing interest in development of automatic segmentation algorithms, which can provide volumetric statistics of whole brain, cortical and subcortical regions, and even substructures of the cortical regions including hippocampal subfields, amygdala nuclei, and thalamic nuclei. Algorithms such as FreeSurfer[63] use spatial positioning and imaging contrast to develop probabilistic models for brain regions, which can then be quantified for volume and contrast or used in conjunction with seed-based tractography to study structural connectivity between brain regions. Because of the dependence of these automatic segmentation algorithms on resolution and image contrast, they are likely to benefit from SNR and resolution gains of ultrahigh field imaging.

FUTURE DIRECTIONS AND SUMMARY

The greater sensitivity and resolution afforded by ultrahigh field imaging have translated into promising increases in clinical benefit. Ultrahigh field imaging still faces challenges, particularly those related to reliable image quality such as B_1 field inhomogeneity. As strategies such as adiabatic pulses and parallel transmission emerge to address these challenges, the case for clinical adoption of this more sensitive technology becomes more straightforward.

Epilepsy, in particular, stands to benefit from these sensitivity benefits in the detection of subtle imaging features that may not be apparent at clinically standard field strengths. These features may provide biomarkers to improve the characterization of this highly heterogeneous disorder and facilitate techniques including deep brain stimulation and resective surgery to provide treatment in cases where noninvasive therapy proves ineffective.

CLINICS CARE POINTS

- Structural images of epileptogenic lesions with an in-plane resolution well under 1 mm can be achieved.
- High resolution, high contrast structural imaging sequences, such as SWI and T2TSE can improve visualization of cortical malformations related to epilepsy.
- Visualization of PVSs in images acquired at 7T is common, and not necessarily an indicator of epilepsy. The distribution, rather than quantity of PVSs may be relevant.
- B1-inhomogeniety, if not carefully managed, my result in images with uneven, dark, or low-contrast areas.
- Sequences requiring high power, such as T2TSE, and FLAIR, may need modification to avoid exceeding SAR-limits.

ACKNOWLEDGMENTS

The authors would like to acknowledge Rebecca Feldman, PhD for her scientific contributions to this chapter.
Dr. Priti Balchandani would like to acknowledge funding from the following sources:
NIH-NINDS R00 NS070821/United States
R01 CA202911/CA/NCI NIH HHS/United States
R01 MH109544/MH/NIMH NIH HHS/United States

DISCLOSURE

Dr. Priti Balchandani (the Principal Investigator in this study) is a named inventor on patents relating to magnetic resonance imaging (MRI) and RF pulse design. The patents have been licensed to GE Healthcare, Siemens AG, and Philips international. Dr. Balchandani receives royalty payments relating to these patents. Dr. Balchandani and Dr. Rebecca Feldman are named inventors on patents relating to Slice-selective adiabatic magnetization T2-preparation (SAMPA) for efficient T2-weighted imaging at ultrahigh field strengths, Methods for Producing a Semi-Adiabatic Spectral-Spatial Spectroscopic Imaging Sequence and Devices Thereof, and Semi-Adiabatic Spectral-spatial Spectroscopic Imaging. These patents have been filed through Mount Sinai Innovation Partners; they remain unlicensed, there is no discussion to license them in the near future, and there are consequently no royalties revolving around them. The remaining authors have nothing to disclose.

REFERENCES

1. Pohmann R, Speck O, Scheffler K. Signal-to-noise ratio and MR tissue parameters in human brain imaging at 3, 7, and 9.4 tesla using current receive coil arrays. Magn Reson Med 2016;75(2):801–9.
2. Pfrommer A, Henning A. On the superlinear increase of the ultimate intrinsic signal-to-noise ratio with regard to main magnetic field strength in a spherical sample. in 2017 International Conference on Electromagnetics in Advanced Applications (ICEAA). Verona, Italy, September 11-15, 2017. IEEE.
3. Van Der Kolk A, Zwanenburg JJ, Denswil NP, et al. Imaging the intracranial atherosclerotic vessel wall using 7T MRI: initial comparison with histopathology. Am J Neuroradiol 2015;36(4):694–701.
4. Middlebrooks EH, Ver Hoef L, Szaflarski JP. Neuroimaging in epilepsy. Curr Neurol Neurosci Rep 2017; 17(4):32.
5. Bell GS, Neligan A, Sander JW. An unknown quantity—the worldwide prevalence of epilepsy. Epilepsia 2014;55(7):958–62.
6. Spencer SS. Neural networks in human epilepsy: evidence of and implications for treatment. Epilepsia 2002;43(3):219–27.
7. Stefan H, Lopes Da Silva FH. Epileptic neuronal networks: methods of identification and clinical relevance. Front Neurol 2013;4:8.
8. Laxer KD, Trinka E, Hirsch LJ, et al. The consequences of refractory epilepsy and its treatment. Epilepsy Behav 2014;37:59–70.
9. Fang M, Xi ZQ, Wu Y, et al. A new hypothesis of drug refractory epilepsy: neural network hypothesis. Med Hypotheses 2011;76(6):871–6.
10. Bernasconi N, Natsume J, Bernasconi A. Progression in temporal lobe epilepsy: differential atrophy in mesial temporal structures. Neurology 2005; 65(2):223–8.
11. Tosun D, Dabbs K, Caplan R, et al. Deformation-based morphometry of prospective neurodevelopmental changes in new onset paediatric epilepsy. Brain 2011;134(Pt 4):1003–14.

12. Coan A, Appenzeller S, Bonilha L, et al. Seizure frequency and lateralization affect progression of atrophy in temporal lobe epilepsy. Neurology 2009; 73(11):834–42.

13. Bonilha L, Rorden C, Appenzeller S, et al. Gray matter atrophy associated with duration of temporal lobe epilepsy. Neuroimage 2006;32(3):1070–9.

14. Fuerst D, Shah J, Kupsky WJ, et al. Volumetric MRI, pathological, and neuropsychological progression in hippocampal sclerosis. Neurology 2001;57(2): 184–8.

15. Bernhardt BC, Worsley KJ, Kim H, et al. Longitudinal and cross-sectional analysis of atrophy in pharmacoresistant temporal lobe epilepsy. Neurology 2009;72(20):1747–54.

16. Briellmann RS, Berkovic SF, Syngeniotis A, et al. Seizure-associated hippocampal volume loss: a longitudinal magnetic resonance study of temporal lobe epilepsy. Ann Neurol 2002;51(5):641–4.

17. Cendes F. Progressive hippocampal and extrahippocampal atrophy in drug resistant epilepsy. Curr Opin Neurol 2005;18(2):173–7.

18. Sidhu MK, Duncan JS, Sander JW. Neuroimaging in epilepsy. Curr Opin Neurol 2018;31(4):371–8.

19. McDonald CR, Hagler DJ, Ahmadi ME, et al. Subcortical and cerebellar atrophy in mesial temporal lobe epilepsy revealed by automatic segmentation. Epilepsy Res 2008;79(2–3):130–8.

20. Feldman RE, Rutland JW, Fields MC, et al. Quantification of perivascular spaces at 7T: A potential MRI biomarker for epilepsy. Seizure 2018;54:11–8.

21. Wuerfel J, Haertle M, Waiczies H, et al. Perivascular spaces—MRI marker of inflammatory activity in the brain? Brain 2008;131(Pt 9):2332–40.

22. Balchandani P, Naidich T. Ultra-high-field MR neuroimaging. AJNR Am J Neuroradiol 2015;36(7): 1204–15.

23. Liao W, Zhang Z, Pan Z, et al. Altered functional connectivity and small-world in mesial temporal lobe epilepsy. PLoS One 2010;5(1):e8525.

24. Waites AB, Briellmann RS, Saling MM, et al. Functional connectivity networks are disrupted in left temporal lobe epilepsy. Ann Neurol 2006;59(2):335–43.

25. Rutland JW, Feldman RE, Delman BN, et al. Subfield-specific tractography of the hippocampus in epilepsy patients at 7 Tesla. Seizure 2018;62:3–10.

26. Cukiert A, Cukiert CM, Argentoni-Baldochi M, et al. Intraoperative neurophysiological responses in epileptic patients submitted to hippocampal and thalamic deep brain stimulation. Seizure 2011; 20(10):748–53.

27. Brown SSG, Rutland JW, Verma G, et al. Ultra-High-Resolution Imaging of Amygdala Subnuclei Structural Connectivity in Major Depressive Disorder. Biol Psychiatry Cogn Neurosci Neuroimaging 2020; 5(2):184–93.

28. Brown S, Rutland JW, Verma G, et al. Structural MRI at 7T reveals amygdala nuclei and hippocampal subfield volumetric association with major depressive disorder symptom severity. Sci Rep 2019;9(1): 1–10.

29. Elder C, Friedman D, Devinsky O, et al. Responsive neurostimulation targeting the anterior nucleus of the thalamus in 3 patients with treatment-resistant multifocal epilepsy. Epilepsia Open 2019;4(1):187–92.

30. Abosch A, Yacoub E, Ugurbil K, et al. An assessment of current brain targets for deep brain stimulation surgery with susceptibility-weighted imaging at 7 tesla. Neurosurgery 2010;67(6):1745–56.

31. Duncan JS. Imaging in the surgical treatment of epilepsy. Nat Rev Neurol 2010;6(10):537.

32. Tracy JI, Doucet GE. Resting-state functional connectivity in epilepsy: growing relevance for clinical decision making. Curr Opin Neurol 2015;28(2): 158–65.

33. He X, Doucet GE, Sperling M, et al. Reduced thalamocortical functional connectivity in temporal lobe epilepsy. Epilepsia 2015;56(10):1571–9.

34. Zhang Z, Liao W, Chen H, et al. Altered functional–structural coupling of large-scale brain networks in idiopathic generalized epilepsy. Brain 2011;134(Pt 10):2912–28.

35. Liao W, Zhang Z, Pan Z, et al. Default mode network abnormalities in mesial temporal lobe epilepsy: a study combining fMRI and DTI. Hum Brain Mapp 2011;32(6):883–95.

36. Duncan JS, Winston GP, Koepp MJ, et al. Brain imaging in the assessment for epilepsy surgery. Lancet Neurol 2016;15(4):420–33.

37. Kuznieck R. Clinical applications of MR spectroscopy in epilepsy. Neuroimaging Clin N Am 2004; 14(3):507–16.

38. Woermann FG, McLean MA, Bartlett PA, et al. Short echo time single-voxel 1H magnetic resonance spectroscopy in magnetic resonance imaging–negative temporal lobe epilepsy: Different biochemical profile compared with hippocampal sclerosis. Ann Neurol 1999;45(3):369–76.

39. Pan JW, Lo KM, Hetherington HP. Role of very high order and degree B0 shimming for spectroscopic imaging of the human brain at 7 tesla. Magn Reson Med 2012;68(4):1007–17.

40. O'Muircheartaigh J, Vollmar C, Traynor C, et al. Clustering probabilistic tractograms using independent component analysis applied to the thalamus. Neuroimage 2011;54(3):2020–32.

41. Vadera S, Mullin J, Bulacio J, et al. Stereoelectroencephalography following subdural grid placement for difficult to localize epilepsy. Neurosurgery 2013; 72(5):723–9.

42. Jayakar P, Gotman J, Harvey AS, et al. Diagnostic utility of invasive EEG for epilepsy surgery:

indications, modalities, and techniques. Epilepsia 2016;57(11):1735–47.

43. Guye M, Bartolomei F, Ranjeva JP. Malformations of cortical development: The role of 7-Tesla magnetic resonance imaging in diagnosis. Rev Neurol (Paris) 2019;175(3):157–62.

44. Sudhyadhom A, Haq IU, Foote KD, et al. A high resolution and high contrast MRI for differentiation of subcortical structures for DBS targeting: the Fast Gray Matter Acquisition T1 Inversion Recovery (FGATIR). Neuroimage 2009;47 Suppl 2:T44–52.

45. Morrison L, Akers A. Cerebral Cavernous Malformation, Familial. 2003 Feb 24 [Updated 2016 Aug 4]. In: Adam MP, Ardinger HH, Pagon RA, et al, editors. GeneReviews® [Internet]. Seattle (WA): University of Washington, Seattle; 1993-2020.

46. Pittau F, Baud MO, Jorge J, et al. MP2RAGE and susceptibility-weighted imaging in lesional epilepsy at 7T. J Neuroimaging 2018;28(4):365–9.

47. Sun K, Cui J, Wang B, et al. Magnetic resonance imaging of tuberous sclerosis complex with or without epilepsy at 7 T. Neuroradiology 2018;60(8):785–94.

48. Feldman RE, Delman BN, Pawha PS, et al. 7T MRI in epilepsy patients with previously normal clinical MRI exams compared against healthy controls. PLoS One 2019;14(3):e0213642.

49. O'Halloran R, Feldman R, Marcuse L, et al. A method for u-fiber quantification from 7T diffusion-weighted MRI data tested in subjects with non-lesional focal epilepsy. Neuroreport 2017; 28(8):457.

50. Chen W, Ogawa S. 10 Principles of BOLD Functional MRI. Red 1999;10:1.

51. Strangman G, Culver JP, Thompson JH, et al. A quantitative comparison of simultaneous BOLD fMRI and NIRS recordings during functional brain activation. Neuroimage 2002;17(2):719–31.

52. Morris LS, Kundu P, Costi S, et al. Ultra-high field MRI reveals mood-related circuit disturbances in depression: A comparison between 3-Tesla and 7-Tesla. Transl Psychiatry 2019;9(1):94.

53. Shah P, Bassett DS, Wisse LEM, et al. Structural and functional asymmetry of medial temporal subregions in unilateral temporal lobe epilepsy: A 7T MRI study. Hum Brain Mapp 2019;40(8):2390–8.

54. Stephenson MC, Gunner F, Napolitano A, et al. Applications of multi-nuclear magnetic resonance spectroscopy at 7T. World J Radiol 2011;3(4):105.

55. Verma G, Hariharan H, Nagarajan R, et al. Implementation of two-dimensional L-COSY at 7 tesla: An investigation of reproducibility in human brain. J Magn Reson Imaging 2014;40(6):1319–27.

56. Terpstra M, Cheong I, Lyu T, et al. Test-retest reproducibility of neurochemical profiles with short-echo, single-voxel MR spectroscopy at 3T and 7T. Magn Reson Med 2016;76(4):1083–91.

57. Feldman RE, Balchandani P. A semiadiabatic spectral-spatial spectroscopic imaging (SASSI) sequence for improved high-field MR spectroscopic imaging. Magn Reson Med 2016;76(4):1071–82.

58. Pan JW, Kuzniecky RI. Utility of magnetic resonance spectroscopic imaging for human epilepsy. Quant Imaging Med Surg 2015;5(2):313.

59. Pan JW, Duckrow RB, Gerrard J, et al. 7T MR spectroscopic imaging in the localization of surgical epilepsy. Epilepsia 2013;54(9):1668–78.

60. Avdievich N, Pan JW, Baehring JM, et al. Short echo spectroscopic imaging of the human brain at 7T using transceiver arrays. Magn Reson Med 2009; 62(1):17–25.

61. Voets NL, Hodgetts CJ, Sen A, et al. Hippocampal MRS and subfield volumetry at 7T detects dysfunction not specific to seizure focus. Sci Rep 2017;7(1): 1–14.

62. Colon A, van Osch MJ, Buijs M, et al. Detection superiority of 7 T MRI protocol in patients with epilepsy and suspected focal cortical dysplasia. Acta Neurol Belg 2016;116(3):259–69.

63. Fischl B. FreeSurfer. Neuroimage 2012;62(2): 774–81.

64. Yushkevich PA, Wang H, Pluta J, et al. Nearly automatic segmentation of hippocampal subfields in in vivo focal T2-weighted MRI. Neuroimage 2010; 53(4):1208–24.

65. Wisse LE, Kuijf HJ, Honingh AM, et al. Automated hippocampal subfield segmentation at 7T MRI. AJNR Am J Neuroradiol 2016;37(6):1050–7.

66. Schoene-Bake JC, Keller SS, Niehusmann P, et al. In vivo mapping of hippocampal subfields in mesial temporal lobe epilepsy: relation to histopathology. Hum Brain Mapp 2014;35(9):4718–28.

67. Santyr BG, Goubran M, Lau JC, et al. Investigation of hippocampal substructures in focal temporal lobe epilepsy with and without hippocampal sclerosis at 7T. J Magn Reson Imaging 2017;45(5): 1359–70.

68. Coras R, Milesi G, Zucca I, et al. 7T MRI features in control human hippocampus and hippocampal sclerosis: an ex vivo study with histologic correlations. Epilepsia 2014;55(12):2003–16.

69. Henry TR, Chupin M, Lehéricy S, et al. Hippocampal sclerosis in temporal lobe epilepsy: findings at 7 T. Radiology 2011;261(1):199–209.

70. Breyer T, Wanke I, Maderwald S, et al. Imaging of patients with hippocampal sclerosis at 7 Tesla: initial results. Acad Radiol 2010;17(4):421–6.

71. De Ciantis A, Barkovich AJ, Cosottini M, et al. Ultra-high-field MR imaging in polymicrogyria and epilepsy. Am J Neuroradiol 2015;36(2):309–16.

72. Wrede KH, Johst S, Dammann P, et al. Caudal image contrast inversion in MPRAGE at 7 Tesla: problem and solution. Acad Radiol 2012;19(2):172–8.

73. Balchandani P, Pauly J, Spielman D. Designing adiabatic radio frequency pulses using the Shinnar–Le Roux algorithm. Magn Reson Med 2010;64(3): 843–51.

74. Balchandani P, Qiu D. Semi-adiabatic Shinnar–Le Roux pulses and their application to diffusion tensor imaging of humans at 7T. Magn Reson Imaging 2014;32(7):804–12.

75. Gumbrecht R, Joonsung L, Fautz H, et al. Fast high-flip pTx pulse design to mitigate B11 inhomogeneity using composite pulses at 7T. Proc Intl Soc Mag Reson Med 2010. Stockholm, Sweden, May 1-7, 2010.

76. O'Brien KR, Magill AW, Delacoste J, et al. Dielectric pads and low- B1+ adiabatic pulses: complementary techniques to optimize structural T1 w whole-brain MP2RAGE scans at 7 tesla. J Magn Reson Imaging 2014;40(4):804–12.

77. Teeuwisse WM, Brink WM, Haines KN, et al. Simulations of high permittivity materials for 7T neuroimaging and evaluation of a new barium titanate-based dielectric. Magn Reson Med 2012;67(4):912–8.

78. Zelinski AC, Angelone LM, Goyal VK, et al. Specific absorption rate studies of the parallel transmission of inner-volume excitations at 7T. J Magn Reson Imaging 2008;28(4):1005–18.

79. Boon P, Vonck K, De Herdt V, et al. Deep brain stimulation in patients with refractory temporal lobe epilepsy. Epilepsia 2007;48(8):1551–60.

80. Lega BC, Halpern CH, Jaggi JL, et al. Deep brain stimulation in the treatment of refractory epilepsy: update on current data and future directions. Neurobiol Dis 2010;38(3):354–60.

81. Charbades S, Kahane P, Minotti L, et al. Deep brain stimulation in epilepsy with particular reference to the subthalamic nucleus. Epileptic Disord 2002;4: S83–93.

82. Akram H, Dayal V, Mahlknecht P, et al. Connectivity derived thalamic segmentation in deep brain stimulation for tremor. Neuroimage Clin 2018;18:130–42.

83. Pouratian N, Zheng Z, Bari AA, et al. Multi-institutional evaluation of deep brain stimulation targeting using probabilistic connectivity-based thalamic segmentation. J Neurosurg 2011;115(5):995–1004.

84. Traynor C, Heckemann RA, Hammers A, et al. Reproducibility of thalamic segmentation based on probabilistic tractography. Neuroimage 2010;52(1): 69–85.

85. Ziyan U, Tuch D, Westin C.-F. Segmentation of thalamic nuclei from DTI using spectral clustering. In International Conference on Medical Image Computing and Computer-Assisted Intervention. Copenhagen, Denmark, October 1-6, 2006. Springer.

86. Wiegell MR, Tuch DS, Larsson HB, et al. Automatic segmentation of thalamic nuclei from diffusion tensor magnetic resonance imaging. NeuroImage 2003;19(2 Pt 1):391–401.

High-Resolution Neurovascular Imaging at 7T

Arterial Spin Labeling Perfusion, 4-Dimensional MR Angiography, and Black Blood MR Imaging

Xingfeng Shao, PhD[a], Lirong Yan, PhD[a,b], Samantha J. Ma, PhD[a,c],
Kai Wang, BS[a], Danny J.J. Wang, PhD, MSCE[a,b],*

KEYWORDS

- Arterial spin labeling (ASL) • Perfusion • Cortical layer • 4-Dimensional MR angiography (4D MRA)
- Lenticulostriate arteries (LSA) • Turbo spin-echo with variable flip angles (TSE VFA)
- Black blood MR imaging

KEY POINTS

- Ultrahigh field offers increased resolution and contrast for neurovascular imaging.
- Ultrahigh field arterial spin labeling has dual benefits of increased signal-to-noise ratio and tracer half-life.
- High-resolution 7T arterial spin labeling allows layer dependent perfusion imaging.
- Four-dimensional MR angiography at 7T provides a detailed visualization of the vascular architecture and dynamic blood flow pattern.
- Black blood MR imaging at 7T allows characterization of small perforating arteries such as lenticulostriate arteries.

INTRODUCTION

Neurovascular imaging at ultrahigh field (UHF) benefits from a high intrinsic signal-to-noise ratio (SNR), which can be leveraged to yield higher spatial resolution and/or higher contrast-to-noise ratio.[1,2] The ability to visualize fine vasculature <1 mm in diameter on clinical standard (1.5T) and high-field (3T) MR imaging is usually limited, whereas UHF ($\geq$7T) MR imaging enables the evaluation of cerebrovascular lesions and vasculature in the neocortex on a submillimeter scale. UHF MR imaging is particularly beneficial to non–contrast-enhanced MR angiography (MRA) and arterial spin labeling (ASL) perfusion with the prolonged T1 of arterial blood at higher field strength. Black blood imaging techniques also benefit from UHF with the ability to achieve isotropic submillimeter resolution, allowing the depiction of smaller perforating arteries, which are critical to characterizing cerebrovascular disease, such as cerebral vasculitis and cerebral autosomal-dominant arteriopathy with subcortical infarcts and leukoencephalopathy.[3–6] Thus, the advent of 7T has resulted in a

[a] Laboratory of FMRI Technology (LOFT), USC Mark & Mary Stevens Neuroimaging and Informatics Institute, Keck School of Medicine, University of Southern California, 2025 Zonal Avenue, Los Angeles, CA 90033, USA; [b] Department of Neurology, Keck School of Medicine, University of Southern California, 2025 Zonal Avenue, Los Angeles, CA 90033, USA; [c] Siemens Healthcare, Los Angeles, CA, USA
* Corresponding author. Laboratory of FMRI Technology (LOFT), Mark & Mary Stevens Neuroimaging and Informatics Institute, Keck School of Medicine, University of Southern California (USC), Los Angeles, CA 90033.
E-mail address: jwang71@gmail.com

Magn Reson Imaging Clin N Am 29 (2021) 53–65
https://doi.org/10.1016/j.mric.2020.09.003
1064-9689/21/© 2020 Elsevier Inc. All rights reserved.

wave of research during the past decade exploring new developments in cerebrovascular imaging, which are now increasingly finding their way into clinical practice.

High-resolution neurovascular imaging is also important to understanding brain function and vasculature in the cortical layers. The pial arteries distribute blood from larger cerebral arteries to descending arterioles and feed capillaries in different cortical layers. After blood passes the capillary space, it is collected by ascending venules and returns to pial veins toward the cortical surface.[7] Blood oxygen level–dependent (BOLD) fMR imaging can achieve submillimeter spatial resolution for studying human brain function at the level of cortical layers and columns at UHF.[8–10] However, the BOLD signal is the result of complex interplays between cerebral blood flow (CBF), cerebral blood volume, and oxygen metabolism, resulting in limited fidelity for inferring the underlying neuronal activation. In addition, the BOLD signal is susceptible to venous contaminations such as the pial veins on the cortical surface that confounds laminar/columnar functional MR imaging (fMR imaging).[9,11–13] High-resolution neurovascular imaging, such as ASL perfusion, is less affected by pial vessels, and thus is crucial to understanding the neurovascular coupling between neuronal activity and ensuing hemodynamic responses.[14]

High-resolution non–contrast-enhanced MRA at UHF enables the precise depiction of cerebral vasculature including both large and small arteries, even arterioles. Time of flight (TOF) has been recognized as a mainstay for evaluating intracranial arteries. With an increased intrinsic SNR and prolonged T1 at UHF, submillimeter resolution TOF (<500 μm) at 7T has been demonstrated,[15,16] with superior angiographic contrast as a result of stronger suppression of stationary background tissue. Recently developed ASL based time-resolved 4-dimensional (4D) MRA[17,18] is another bright blood MRA technique, that allows for the adequate depiction of both vascular structure and dynamic flow patterns. UHF provides sufficient SNR for 4D MRA, which could further benefit the characterization of dynamic flow patterns in cerebrovascular disorders, such as arteriovenous malformation (AVM).[17,19] High-resolution black blood MR imaging was originally developed for imaging extracranial (carotid bifurcation), intracranial vessel arterial wall lesions (including atherosclerotic plaques), and intracranial arterial stenosis.[20–22] The increased SNR at 7T leads to an overall better visualization of the cerebral small vessels, such as lenticulostriate arteries (LSAs) and potentially illustrates the effects of aging and/or vascular risk factors such as hypertension, hyperlipidemia, and diabetes on the vessel structures.[23]

In this article, we focus on the technical developments and emerging clinical and neuroscientific applications of ASL perfusion, 4D MRA, and T1-weighted black blood MR imaging at UHF. Experience with parallel radiofrequency (RF) transmission (pTx) technologies at 7T, which benefit all the above techniques, is also presented. Limitations and challenges such as the specific absorption rate (SAR) and field inhomogeneity are also discussed.

A SHORT OVERVIEW OF PARALLEL RADIOFREQUENCY TRANSMISSION TECHNOLOGY AT 7T

One key technical advance allowing high-resolution neurovascular imaging at UHF is pTx. Currently, the conventional homogeneous birdcage type coil driven by a single RF-pulse waveform, also known as single RF transmission (1Tx), does not possess spatial degrees of freedom and works best for uniform excitations. Although useable at 3T or lower field strengths, nonuniformities arise when the wavelength of the RF waveform approaches the dimensions of the human head. Such effects are observed when imaging at UHF and result in destructive excitation field interference or shading with a characteristic strong center brightening. To mitigate these B1 inhomogeneities, pTx has been proposed as an effective solution. The most common approach for pTx is static RF shimming,[24] where all the transmit channels emit identical RF waveforms with scaled amplitudes and shifted phases. Because pTx enables more spatial degrees of freedom, tailored RF pulses or shape-specific B1 shimming can be implemented to achieve a more uniform B1 field.[25,26]

The latest 7T MAGNETOM Terra system (Siemens Healthineers, Erlangen, Germany) with the 8-channel pTx system and 8Tx/32Rx head coil (Nova Medical, Inc., Wilmington, MA) offers 3 static B1 shim modes to correct B1 inhomogeneities including TrueForm, patient-specific, and volume-selective shimming. The TrueForm shim mode uses 45° phase increments for each adjacent transmit channel to mimic the 1Tx circularly polarized coil. Owing to the increased spatial coverage with the pTx coil geometry, TrueForm shimming with the pTx system can already achieve improved RF uniformity in the temporal and subcortical brain regions compared with 1Tx. In the patient-specific shim mode, the RF excitation is parameterized relative to the B1 maps of the registered subject. This method is optimized for B1 shimming of the whole volume specified by the slice group. Last, the volume-selective shim mode optimizes the B1 field to a specific volume chosen by the user, which is often helpful for improving the homogeneity in an anatomically specific region of interest.[27] Compared with acquisition with 1Tx, the use of pTx significantly improves the RF uniformity across the brain tissue (**Fig. 1**A), leading to a higher SNR in the temporal and subcortical regions (**Fig. 1**B) and ultimately supporting high-resolution imaging across the whole brain at UHF.

ARTERIAL SPIN-LABELED PERFUSION AT 7T

CBF or perfusion measured by ASL is a key parameter for the in vivo assessment of neurovascular function. The ASL signal is close to the site of neural activation, because most of the labeled arterial water exchanges with tissue water in capillaries.[28] It has been shown that ASL perfusion fMR imaging is able to visualize orientation columns in the cat visual cortex with superior spatial resolution compared with BOLD fMR imaging.[29] The hemodynamic response of perfusion signals has also been shown to arise approximately 1 second earlier than that of BOLD signals.[30] Unlike BOLD fMR imaging that detects relative signal changes between 2 conditions, ASL provides quantitative perfusion measurements both at rest and during task activation. UHF ASL has the dual benefits of increased SNR that scales with B0 field and prolonged tracer half-life (blood T1),[31] therefore, it may overcome the major limitation of ASL in terms of low SNR. **Fig. 2**A shows a more than 3-fold SNR gain for 7T ASL compared with 3T ASL predicted by theory. Indeed, our experimental data using turbo-FLASH–based ASL at 7T demonstrated the feasibility of perfusion imaging with near submillimeter spatial resolution, which is not feasible at 3T (**Fig. 2**B).[32]

To achieve whole-brain high-resolution perfusion imaging at 7T, we have recently taken advantage of the 8Tx/32Rx head coil with TrueForm B1 shimming mode on the 7T Terra system, which allowed the application of pseudocontinuous ASL (pCASL) at the base of the brain.[33] In addition, a novel time-dependent 2D controlled aliasing in parallel imaging results in higher acceleration technique[34] was implemented in a 3D gradient and spin echo sequence to achieve a robust high-resolution and highly accelerated 3D imaging (up to 12-fold) by efficiently exploiting coil sensitivity variations along both phase and slice dimensions (lower coil g-factor), as well as temporal incoherence of sampling patterns across ASL

measurements (**Fig. 3**A).[33] A novel image reconstruction method employing both spatial and temporal total generalized variation regularization[35] was applied to reconstruct high-resolution (2 mm isotropic) CBF maps with nearly whole brain coverage and 12-fold acceleration (**Fig. 3**B). This novel ASL total generalized variation method also had denoising capabilities to minimize effects of head motion and physiologic noise on perfusion images at 7T.

Adiabatic pulses have been commonly used as the inversion pulse for pulsed ASL (PASL) to address the issues of B0 and B1 inhomogeneity at UHF. To improve the quality and accuracy of the perfusion map acquired at 7T, we recently optimized and systematically evaluated 4 commonly used adiabatic inversion pulses including the hyperbolic secant pulse,[36] wideband uniform rate smooth truncation (WURST) pulse,[37] frequency offset correction inversion (FOCI) pulse,[38] and time-resampled FOCI pulse[39] based on a custom-defined loss function that took into account the labeling efficiency and the residual tissue signal.[40] This study again used the 8Tx/32Rx head coil with TrueForm B1 shimming mode on 7T Terra. The perfusion maps of the 4 pulse sequences of 1 representative subject are shown in **Fig. 4**. The optimized WURST pulse achieved a good balance between high labeling efficiency and low residual tissue signal, with higher labeling efficiency than hyperbolic secant and time-resampled FOCI pulses, and lower residual tissue signal than FOCI pulse. The relative labeling efficiency versus residual tissue signal of the WURST PASL sequence was significantly higher than any of the other 3 sequences ($P<.01$ for each case). Furthermore, the PASL sequence with the optimized WURST pulse was able to provide nearly whole brain perfusion imaging at 7T.

LAYER-DEPENDENT PERFUSION IMAGING

Because the thickness of the cerebral cortex is usually less than 3 mm,[41] submillimeter spatial resolution is required to study layer- or depth-dependent structural and/or physiologic changes. Recent research has demonstrated that the pCASL labeling scheme combined with efficient 3D inner-volume gradient and spin echo readout and background suppression has the capability of revealing layer dependent CBF at UHF of 7T.[14] Because the ASL signal is quantitative and originated primarily from capillaries and brain tissue, this new development opens the door to investigating neurovascular coupling with an unprecedented precision at the laminar level.

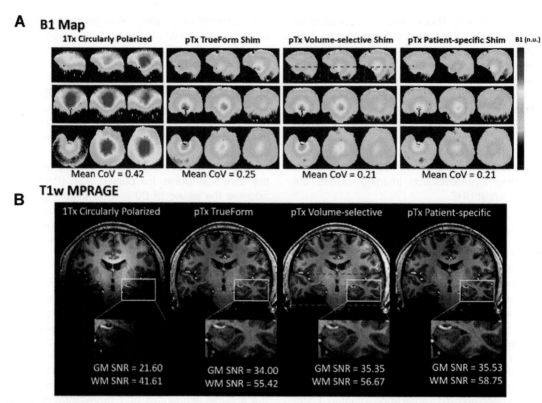

Fig. 1. In vivo comparisons of various coil configurations using either pTx-mode or 1Tx-mode. (*A*) Measured B1+ field distributions in sagittal (*top row*), axial (*middle row*), and coronal (*bottom row*) views. The mean coefficient of variation (CoV = SD/mean) was measured after each B1+ field shimming process. (*B*) Gray matter (GM) and white matter (WM) SNR comparison demonstrating the increased coverage with pTx for T1-weighted MPRAGE images. The pTx patient-specific shimming produced the highest SNR for gray–white matter contrast in the temporal lobe region (*yellow box*). The *red dashed box* indicates the volume prescribed for pTx volume-selective B1 shimming. SD, standard deviation. (*Adapted from* Ma SJ, Zhao C, Wang K, et al. Anatomical NeuroImaging with Single and Parallel Transmission at Ultra-high Field: A Comparison of Image Quality and User Experience. Intl Soc Mag Reson Med. 2020;Vol 28. With permission.)

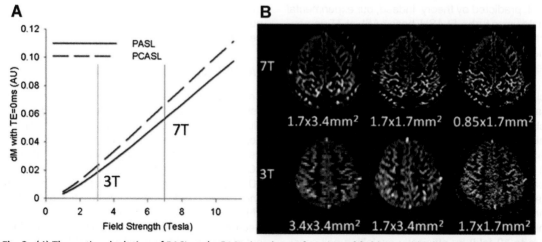

Fig. 2. (*A*) Theoretic calculation of PASL and pCASL signals as a function of field strength, showing a greater than 3-fold SNR gain from 3T to 7T. (*B*) pCASL perfusion images at 7T and 3T with 3 different resolutions. AU, arbitrary units. (*Adapted from* Zuo Z, Wang R, Zhuo Y, et al. Turbo-FLASH based arterial spin labeled perfusion MRI at 7 T. PloS one. 2013;8(6). With permission.)

A 2D CAIPI under-sampling pattern for 12-fold acceleration

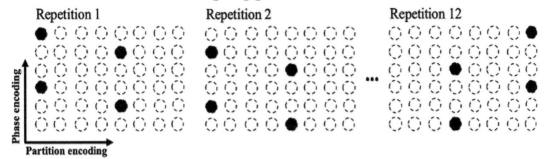

B Whole-brain CBF map with ~2 mm isotropic resolution

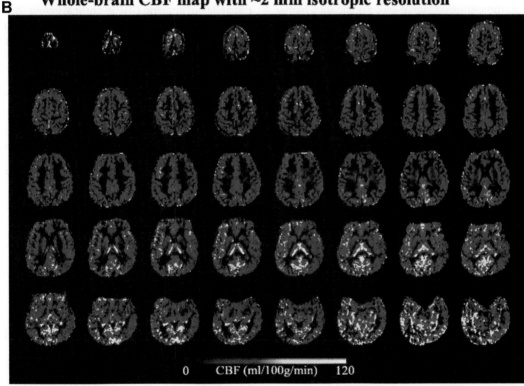

0   CBF (ml/100g/min)   120

Fig. 3. (*A*) Implementation of the time-dependent 2D CAIPI undersampling pattern. The acceleration factor is 3 along phase encoding direction and 4 along the partition-encoding direction. The total acceleration factor is 12. The acceleration pattern is shifted between repetitions along phase/partition encoding direction to increase the temporal incoherence. (*B*) Whole brain CBF map acquired with 2D-CAIPI acquisition and spatial/temporal total generalized variation reconstruction. CAIPIA, controlled aliasing in volumetric parallel. (*Adapted from* Shao X, Spann SM, Wang K, et al. High-resolution whole brain ASL perfusion imaging at 7T with 12-fold acceleration and spatial-temporal regularized reconstruction. Intl Soc Mag Reson Med. 2020;Vol 28. With permission.)

Fig. 5 shows submillimeter multidelay perfusion images (B) and a CBF map (C) acquired from one healthy subject (female, 38 years old) using pCASL with a background-suppressed 3D inner-volume gradient and spin echo at 7T. The labeling plane was applied above the circle of Willis and 50 mm below the center of the imaging volume (left motor cortex) using the 1Tx/32Rx coil. The in-plane resolution was 0.5 mm after interpolation, and slice thickness was 1.4 mm. Three layers of gray matter (superficial, middle, and deep) were manually segmented based on co-registered T1w MPRAGE images. **Fig. 5D** and E show the bar plot of multidelay perfusion signals and CBF values averaged from 4 participants (2 male and 2 female, 31.5 ± 3.1 years

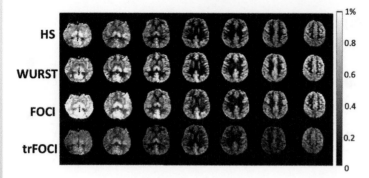

Fig. 4. Perfusion map acquired using the optimized adiabatic inversion pulses. For hyperbolic secant (HS) and FOCI, the residual tissue signal is dominant at bottom slices. The mean gray matter perfusion is 0.42%, 0.60%, 0.59%, and 0.35% for HS, WURST, FOCI, and time-resampled FOCI, respectively. (*Adapted from* Wang K, Shao X, Yan L, et al. Optimization of adiabatic pulses for Pulsed ASL at 7T – Comparison with Pseudo-continuous ASL. Proc ISMRM 2020;28:3695; with permission.)

old). The perfusion signal was significantly higher in the middle layer than the superficial or deep layer (approximately 20%) at a post-labeling delay (PLD) of 1000 ms and 1500 ms (*P*<.05). The average CBF was 42.1, 49.4, and 40.3 mL/100 g/min in the superficial, middle, and deep layers, respectively. The CBF was significantly higher in the middle layer (approximately 20%; *P*<.001), which matches well with the highest capillary density observed in the middle layers as reported in anatomic studies in animals and specimens of human brain tissue.[42] The

capability of imaging CBF in cortical layers allows new opportunities for investigating the microvascular blood supply and neurovascular coupling in a laminar fashion.

FOUR-DIMENSIONAL MR ANGIOGRAPHY AT 7T

Besides tissue perfusion or CBF, ASL also offers angiographic contrast. With a shorter postlabeling delay time after ASL preparation, the majority of labeled blood is still within arteries; thus, an MRA

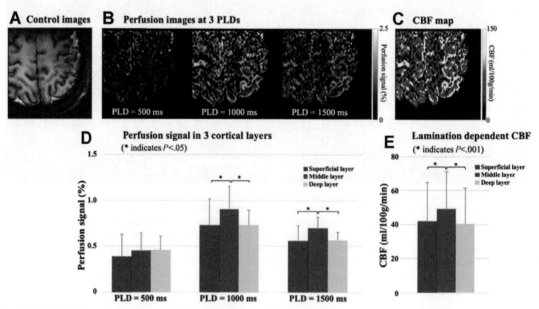

Fig. 5. Multidelay perfusion images (*B*) and CBF maps (*C*) with submillimeter in-plane resolution (0.5 mm, after interpolation) acquired at 7T. (*A*) The corresponding structural control images. A small field of view was acquired using inner-volume 3D gradient and spin echo readout to shorten the acquisition time and increase the SNR. (*D*) A bar plot of the perfusion signal (normalized by M0) at a post-labeling delay (PLD) of 500, 1000, and 1500 ms in 3 layers of the motor cortex. Multidelay perfusion images reveal the dynamic passage of labeled signals, and the majority of labeled spins arrive into capillary space at a PLD of 1000 ms. The perfusion signal in the middle layer is significantly higher (approximately 20%) than the superficial or deep layer at a PLD of 1000 and 1500 ms. (*E*) shows the bar plot of CBF, which was computed by a weighted-delay approach. CBF in the middle layer is 17.3% higher than the superficial layer and 22.7% higher than the deep layer.

is obtained. Over the past decade, a number of studies have applied ASL for MRA purposes by taking advantage of recent advances in both ASL labeling and image acquisition.[17,18,43–49] In particular, an ASL-based time-resolved non–contrast-enhanced 4D MRA has been developed, which offers spatial resolution of approximately 1 mm³ and temporal resolution of 50 to 100 ms.[17,44] This 4D MRA shows potential for characterizing cerebrovascular dynamic flow patterns in cerebrovascular disorders, such as AVM.[19,50,51] However, it remains a challenge to capture the draining vein, which serves as a critical criterion in clinical diagnosis in AVM,[19,50,51] when using 4D MRA at conventional 1.5T and 3T as a result of relatively short trace half-life (blood T1).

The SNR of ASL-based MRA is considerably higher than that of ASL perfusion, given the high concentration of labeled blood within an arterial voxel as well as minimal postlabeling delay time. UHF further benefits ASL-based MRA with increased intrinsic SNR and prolonged blood T1. Therefore, 4D MRA at 7T allows for detailed characterization of vascular architecture as well as dynamic flow patterns. Our previous work has initially demonstrated the feasibility of 4D MRA at 7T using both standard 3D Cartesian acquisition and advanced non-Cartesian acquisition with golden angle stack-of-stars radial sampling.[52] **Fig. 6** shows 6 selected temporal frames of 4D MRA with a spatial resolution of isotropic 1 mm and temporal resolution of 96 ms collected on a 7T

Terra from a healthy volunteer using the 1Tx/32Rx head coil. One can appreciate the fine vascular structures as well as dynamic blood flow through the cerebral vasculature. A 4D MRA at 7T also shows improved delineation of AVM features, especially the draining veins. **Fig. 7** shows a comparison of 4D MRA at 3T and 7T for an AVM case. We can clearly observe the labeled blood flow through the feeding arteries and nidus on both 3T and 7T, matching the digital subtraction angiography findings nicely. However, the draining vein can only be clearly visualized at 7T owing to the prolonged blood T1, although it failed to be visible at 3T. Therefore, 7T possesses potential clinical utility (and advantage over 3T) in the evaluation of AVMs and other cerebrovascular diseases with slow flow.

BLACK BLOOD MR IMAGING AT 7T

High-resolution black blood MR imaging is a recent technique originally developed for imaging intracranial vessel wall and plaque using 3D T1-weighted turbo spin echo (TSE) sequences with variable flip angles (VFA).[53–55] The technique has previously been implemented on various platforms and field strengths, allowing the potential for straightforward translation to clinical imaging. Particularly at UHF, the long echo train of the TSE technique offers 3 advantages for visualizing small vessels: (1) adequate flow suppression by inherent dephasing of flowing signals (black blood

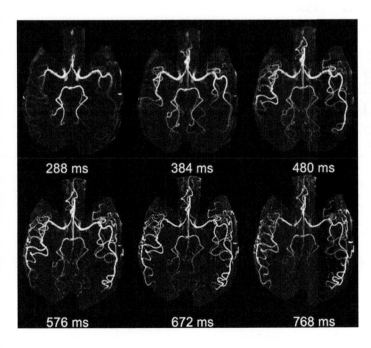

Fig. 6. An example of 4D MRA using 3D Cartesian acquisition with a spatial resolution of 1 × 1 × 1 mm³ at 7T. Six representative 4D MRA maximum intensity projection images along the axial direction are displayed. Detailed delineation of dynamic blood flow through cerebral vasculature can be appreciated.

288 ms 384 ms 480 ms

576 ms 672 ms 768 ms

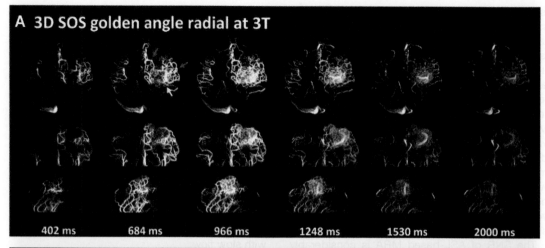

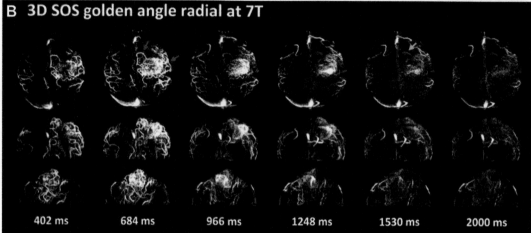

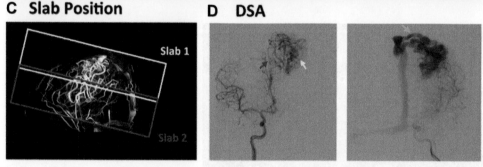

Fig. 7. An AVM case with 2 slabs acquired with 4D MRA using golden-angle stack-of-stars (SOS) radial acquisition at 3T (*A*) and 7T (*B*). Six representative maximum intensity projection images are displayed along axial, coronal, and sagittal views. The positions of the 2 slabs are shown in the TOF image (*C*). Digital subtraction angiography (DSA) images serve as the gold standard (*D*). The entire AVM lesion, including feeding arteries (*red arrow*), nidus (*yellow arrow*), and draining vein (*green arrow*), was captured in a 2-slab radial 4D MRA. The 4D MRA matches well with the DSA image. It can be noted that the draining vein (*green arrow* in *B*) is better depicted at 7T than that at 3T. (*Adapted from* Cong F, Zhuo Y, Yu S, et al. Noncontrast-enhanced time-resolved 4D dynamic intracranial MR angiography at 7T: A feasibility study. J Magn Reson Imaging. 2018;48(1):111-120; with permission.)

MR imaging); (2) high spatial resolution (isotropic 0.5 mm or higher); and (3) near whole-brain coverage in a clinically acceptable time (<10 minutes). In addition to providing improved plaque characterization at the large artery vessel wall,[56] these features suggest that black blood MR imaging is particularly suitable for visualizing cerebral small vessels such as the LSAs and other perforating arteries as well.

Our previous study demonstrated the optimization of the T1-weighted TSE-VFA sequence at UHF for the delineation of LSAs in a healthy cohort.[23] As a comparison, 7T TOF MRA is the reference standard for visualizing and quantifying LSAs.[57] As shown in **Fig. 8**, black blood MR imaging whether at 3T or 7T was able to detect more LSAs likely because the saturation effect of TOF MRA on slow flowing spins led to a compromised delineation of smaller LSAs, usually on the medial side of the middle cerebral artery. Conversely, LSAs can be reliably visualized by T1-weighted TSE-VFA owing to combined effects of longer T1/T2 values of arterial blood and flow-induced phase dispersion during TSE readout at both 3T and 7T. The delineation of LSAs in T1-weighted TSE-VFA images can be a useful tool to evaluate and potentially illustrate the effects of aging and/or vascular risk factors such as hypertension,

hyperlipidemia, and diabetes on the vessel structures. This technique may also be possibly used for the visualization of small hypertensive-related Charcot–Bouchard aneurysms of the LSAs, which can result in catastrophic basal ganglionic hemorrhages. Given the sharpness and improved SNR at UHF, automated or deep learning-based segmentation algorithms can be applied to these high-resolution black blood images to perform a quantitative shape analysis of LSA morphology.[58]

There remain some challenges to address regarding the use of black blood MR imaging for clinical small vessel characterization at UHF. The image contrast of small perforating arteries may be affected by B1 inhomogeneity, especially at UHF. Fortunately, the central location of LSAs at the central bright spot of B1+ field owing to dielectric effects at 7T is favorable for enhancing the contrast-to-noise ratio of LSAs. However, to observe other perforating arteries in the neocortex or larger vessels at the base of the brain, solutions such as pTx shimming should be applied. **Fig. 9** demonstrates the benefit of using pTx B1 shimming for improving detailed delineation of perforating arteries, as well as achieving more homogeneous signal at the base of the brain near the circle of Willis. With the better coverage provided by pTx, we can take full advantage of

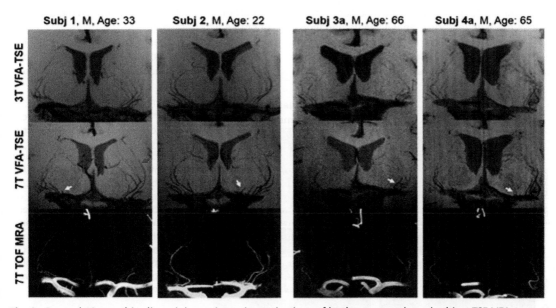

Fig. 8. Coronal 10-mm thin slice minimum intensity projections of both young and aged subject TSE-VFA scans at 3T (*top row*) and 7T (*middle row*). With the increased field strength, the LSAs are more clearly delineated, especially in the distal portions of the vessels (*red arrows*). The bottom row shows a coronal 10-mm thin slice maximum intensity projection of 7T TOF MRA. TSE-VFA can resolve more LSAs than 7T TOF MRA, especially for the LSAs located in the medial group along the middle cerebral artery (*white arrows*). (*Adapted from* Ma SJ, Sarabi MS, Yan L, et al. Characterization of lenticulostriate arteries with high resolution black-blood T1-weighted turbo spin echo with variable flip angles at 3 and 7 Tesla. Neuroimage. 2019;199:184-193; with permission.)

the whole brain, high-resolution features of T1-weighted TSE-VFA for the morphologic evaluation of cerebral vasculature from arteries to very small arterioles.

POTENTIALS AND CHALLENGES OF NEUROVASCULAR IMAGING AT 7T

In this article, we showcase several new developments in neurovascular imaging at 7T, including high-resolution PASL and pCASL with near whole brain coverage, cortical layer–dependent perfusion imaging, 4D time-resolved MRA, and black blood MR imaging. These new techniques have many clinical and neuroscientific applications. For instance, high-resolution ASL at UHF allows the characterization of small cortical lesions in multiple sclerosis that previously could only be imaged using contrast-enhanced MR imaging.[59] The increased SNR and prolonged blood T1 (>2 seconds) at UHF should make it feasible for a reliable measurement of white matter perfusion using ASL, which has been challenging owing to the increased transit time and lower CBF in white matter than in gray matter.[60] The capability for laminar perfusion imaging in human brain is groundbreaking. To date, such information can only be obtained by anatomic studies in animals and specimens of human brain tissue.[42] The laminar profile of resting perfusion may be treated as a surrogate index of microvascular density across the human cortex, as well as its variations with neurodegeneration in Alzheimer's disease and multiple sclerosis. Such information can be incorporated into modeling work to explain depth-dependent BOLD responses.[9] In addition, task activation–induced perfusion changes can be investigated in a layer-dependent fashion without the contamination of pial veins seen in BOLD fMR imaging. Given the tight neurovascular coupling between neuronal activity and microvascular perfusion, our ability to infer underlying neuronal activity in health and disease will be greatly enhanced.

The increased SNR and prolonged T1 at UHF are also highly beneficial for both bright and black blood MRA/MR imaging. As shown in **Fig. 7**, the draining vein of an AVM can only be visualized by 4D MRA at 7T but not at 3T. Black blood MR imaging with T1-weighted TSE-VFA at both 3T and 7T is able to visualize more LSAs than TOF MRA at 7T, and offers concurrent evaluation of vessel wall and parenchymal lesions. Black blood MR imaging at 7T provides sharper delineation of LSAs than 3T, especially in the distal portions of the vessels (see **Fig. 8**). However, the perivascular space also seems to be dark on T1-weighted TSE-VFA images, and the spatial resolution of existing black blood MR imaging does not allow for the differentiation of lumen from perivascular space signals of small vessels. It will be interesting to combine both bright and black blood MRA/MR imaging to fully characterize the morphology and function of small vessels in human brain at UHF. Such capability will be highly appealing for the characterization of cerebral small vessel disease, which is a major cause of stroke and dementia.[61]

The challenges of neurovascular imaging at UHF include B1/B0 field inhomogeneities and SAR constraints. The pTx technology already showed

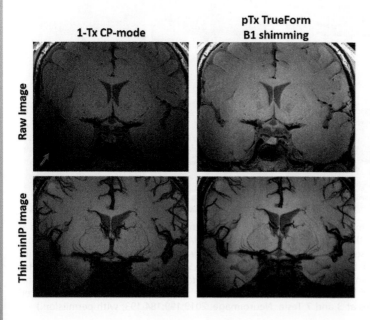

Fig. 9. The LSAs are located in the central "bright spot" of the B1+ field owing to standing wave shading artifacts (dielectric effects, *red arrow*) at 7T, which is favorable for enhancing the contrast-to-noise ratio of LSAs, but problematic for evaluating larger vessels at the base of the brain or perforating arteries in the parenchyma. With the use of pTx B1 shimming, the dielectric effects toward the base of the brain are decreased , improving the overall SNR and enabling concurrent vessel wall assessment.

promise in mitigating B1 field inhomogeneity in our 7T studies, although we only used the basic True-Form shim mode that simulates 1Tx circularly polarized excitation. For the next step, we will compare TrueForm with patient-specific and volume-selective shimming modes, and the latter 2 are expected to yield a more homogeneous B1 field at the cost of a greater level of SAR. For adiabatic inversion pulses, the minimum B1 intensity can be maximized using RF shimming to improve the labeling efficiency.[62] More advanced strategies such as dynamic pTx pulses[63] can be further applied, where each RF channel plays out channel-specific waveforms creating time-dependent spatial interference patterns to reach an ideal tradeoff between B1 field homogeneity and SAR.

SUMMARY

We present several new developments for high-resolution neurovascular imaging at 7T. In conjunction with other technical advances at UHF such as pTx technologies, the suite of new methods can characterize the structure and function of the cerebral vasculature from arteries to arterioles and capillaries with submillimeter spatial resolution.

ACKNOWLEDGMENTS

This work was supported by National Institutes of Health (NIH) grant UH3-NS100614, S10-OD025312, R01-NS114382, R01-EB028297, R01NS118019, K25-AG056594 and American Heart Association (AHA) grant AHA16SDG29630013.

DISCLOSURE

Nothing to disclose.

REFERENCES

1. De Cocker LJ, Lindenholz A; Zwanenburg JJ, et al. Clinical vascular imaging in the brain at 7 T. Neuroimage 2018;168:452–8.
2. Rutland J, Delman B, Gill C, et al. Emerging use of ultra-high-field 7T MRI in the study of intracranial vascularity: state of the field and future directions. AJNR Am J Neuroradiol 2020;41(1):2–9.
3. Bousser MG, Biousse V. Small vessel vasculopathies affecting the central nervous system. J Neuroophthalmol 2004;24(1):56–61.
4. Pantoni L. Cerebral small vessel disease: from pathogenesis and clinical characteristics to therapeutic challenges. Lancet Neurol 2010;9(7):689–701.
5. Pantoni L, Pescini F, Nannucci S, et al. Comparison of clinical, familial, and MRI features of CADASIL
6. and NOTCH3-negative patients. Neurology 2010; 74(1):57–63.
6. Scolding NJ. Central nervous system vasculitis. Semin Immunopathol 2009;31(4):527–36.
7. Schmid F, Barrett MJP, Jenny P, et al. Vascular density and distribution in neocortex. Neuroimage 2019; 197:792–805.
8. Koopmans PJ, Barth M, Orzada S, et al. Multi-echo fMRI of the cortical laminae in humans at 7 T. Neuroimage 2011;56(3):1276–85.
9. Polimeni JR, Fischl B, Greve DN, et al. Laminar analysis of 7 T BOLD using an imposed spatial activation pattern in human V1. Neuroimage 2010;52(4): 1334–46.
10. Cheng K, Waggoner RA, Tanaka K. Human ocular dominance columns as revealed by high-field functional magnetic resonance imaging. Neuron 2001; 32(2):359–74.
11. De Martino F, Zimmermann J, Muckli L, et al. Cortical depth dependent functional responses in humans at 7T: improved specificity with 3D GRASE. PLoS One 2013;8(3):e60514.
12. Yacoub E, Shmuel A, Logothetis N, et al. Robust detection of ocular dominance columns in humans using Hahn Spin Echo BOLD functional MRI at 7 Tesla. Neuroimage 2007;37(4):1161–77.
13. Moerel M, De Martino F, Kemper VG, et al. Sensitivity and specificity considerations for fMRI encoding, decoding, and mapping of auditory cortex at ultra-high field. Neuroimage 2018;164:18–31.
14. Shao X, Wang K, Wang DJ. 7T high-resolution arterial spin labeling reveals layer dependent cerebral blood flow. In. Vol 27. Proceedings of ISMRM 2019; 849.
15. Kang CK, Park CW, Han JY, et al. Imaging and analysis of lenticulostriate arteries using 7.0-Tesla magnetic resonance angiography. Magn Reson Med 2009;61(1):136–44.
16. Zwanenburg JJ, Hendrikse J, Takahara T, et al. MR angiography of the cerebral perforating arteries with magnetization prepared anatomical reference at 7T: comparison with time-of-flight. J Magn Reson Imaging 2008;28(6):1519–26.
17. Yan L, Wang S, Zhuo Y, et al. Unenhanced dynamic MR angiography: high spatial and temporal resolution by using true FISP–based spin tagging with alternating radiofrequency. Radiology 2010;256(1):270–9.
18. Yan L, Salomon N, Wang DJ. Time-resolved noncontrast enhanced 4-D dynamic magnetic resonance angiography using multibolus TrueFISP-based spin tagging with alternating radiofrequency (TrueSTAR). Magn Reson Med 2014;71(2):551–60.
19. Yu S, Yan L, Yao Y, et al. Noncontrast dynamic MRA in intracranial arteriovenous malformation (AVM): comparison with time of flight (TOF) and digital subtraction angiography (DSA). Magn Reson Imaging 2012;30(6):869–77.

20. Zhu C, Haraldsson H, Tian B, et al. High resolution imaging of the intracranial vessel wall at 3 and 7 T using 3D fast spin echo MRI. Magn Reson Mater Phys Biol Med 2016;29(3):559–70.

21. Harteveld AA, van der Kolk AG, van der Worp HB, et al. High-resolution intracranial vessel wall MRI in an elderly asymptomatic population: comparison of 3T and 7T. Eur Radiol 2017;27(4):1585–95.

22. Baradaran H, Patel P, Gialdini G, et al. Quantifying intracranial internal carotid artery stenosis on MR Angiography. AJNR Am J Neuroradiol 2017;38(5): 986–90.

23. Ma SJ, Sarabi MS, Yan L, et al. Characterization of lenticulostriate arteries with high resolution black-blood T1-weighted turbo spin echo with variable flip angles at 3 and 7 Tesla. Neuroimage 2019;199: 184–93.

24. Zhu Y. Parallel excitation with an array of transmit coils. Magn Reson Med 2004;51(4):775–84.

25. Hoult DI, Phil D. Sensitivity and power deposition in a high-field imaging experiment. J Magn Reson Imaging 2000;12(1):46–67.

26. Ibrahim TS, Lee R, Baertlein BA, et al. Application of finite difference time domain method for the design of birdcage RF head coils using multi-port excitations. Magn Reson Imaging 2000;18(6):733–42.

27. TimTX syngo MR E12 operator manual. Erlangen, Germany: Siemens Healthcare GmbH; 2018.

28. Detre JA, Wang J. Technical aspects and utility of fMRI using BOLD and ASL. Clin Neurophysiol 2002;113(5):621–34.

29. Duong TQ, Kim D-S, Uğurbil K, et al. Localized cerebral blood flow response at submillimeter columnar resolution. Proc Natl Acad Sci U S A 2001;98(19):10904–9.

30. Liu HL, Pu Y, Nickerson LD, et al. Comparison of the temporal response in perfusion and BOLD-based event-related functional MRI. Magn Reson Med 2000;43(5):768–72.

31. Wang J, Alsop DC, Li L, et al. Comparison of quantitative perfusion imaging using arterial spin labeling at 1.5 and 4.0 Tesla. Magn Reson Med 2002;48(2): 242–54.

32. Zuo Z, Wang R, Zhuo Y, et al. Turbo-FLASH based arterial spin labeled perfusion MRI at 7 T. PLoS One 2013;8(6):e66612.

33. Shao X, Spann SM, Wang K, Yan L, Rudolf S, Wang DJ. High-resolution whole brain ASL perfusion imaging at 7T with 12-fold acceleration and spatial-temporal regularized reconstruction. In. Vol 28. Proceedings of ISMRM 2020; 23.

34. Breuer FA, Blaimer M, Mueller MF, et al. Controlled aliasing in volumetric parallel imaging (2D CAIPIRINHA). Magn Reson Med 2006;55(3):549–56.

35. Spann SM, Shao X, Wang DJ, et al. Robust single-shot acquisition of high resolution whole brain ASL images by combining time-dependent 2D CAPIRINHA sampling with spatio-temporal TGV reconstruction. Neuroimage 2020;206:116337.

36. Silver M, Joseph R, Hoult D. Highly selective π2 and π pulse generation. J Magn Reson 1969;59(2): 347–51.

37. Kupce E. Adiabatic pulses for wideband inversion and broadband decoupling. J Magn Reson 1995; Series A(115):4.

38. Ordidge RJ, Wylezinska M, Hugg JW, et al. Frequency offset corrected inversion (FOCI) pulses for use in localized spectroscopy. Magn Reson Med 1996;36(4):562–6.

39. Hurley AC, Al-Radaideh A, Bai L, et al. Tailored RF pulse for magnetization inversion at ultrahigh field. Magn Reson Med 2010;63(1):51–8.

40. Wang K, Shao X, Yan L, Jin J, Wang D. Optimization of adiabatic pulses for pulsed ASL at 7T - comparison with pseudo-continuous ASL. Proceedings of ISMRM, Vol 28, 2020; 3695.

41. Tamnes CK, Herting MM, Goddings A-L, et al. Development of the cerebral cortex across adolescence: a multisample study of inter-related longitudinal changes in cortical volume, surface area, and thickness. J Neurosci 2017;37(12):3402–12.

42. Lauwers F, Cassot F, Lauwers-Cances V, et al. Morphometry of the human cerebral cortex microcirculation: general characteristics and space-related profiles. Neuroimage 2008;39(3):936–48.

43. van Osch MJ, Hendrikse J, Golay X, et al. Non-invasive visualization of collateral blood flow patterns of the circle of Willis by dynamic MR angiography. Med image Anal 2006;10(1):59–70.

44. Bi X, Weale P, Schmitt P, et al. Non-contrast-enhanced four-dimensional (4D) intracranial MR angiography: a feasibility study. Magn Reson Med 2010;63(3):835–41.

45. Okell TW, Schmitt P, Bi X, et al. Optimization of 4D vessel-selective arterial spin labeling angiography using balanced steady-state free precession and vessel-encoding. NMR Biomed 2016; 29(6):776–86.

46. Shao X, Zhao Z, Russin J, et al. Quantification of intracranial arterial blood flow using noncontrast enhanced 4D dynamic MR angiography. Magn Reson Med 2019;82(1):449–59.

47. Song HK, Yan L, Smith RX, et al. Noncontrast enhanced four-dimensional dynamic MRA with golden angle radial acquisition and K-space weighted image contrast (KWIC) reconstruction. Magn Reson Med 2014;72(6):1541–51.

48. Zhou Z, Han F, Yu S, et al. Accelerated noncontrast-enhanced 4-dimensional intracranial MR angiography using golden-angle stack-of-stars trajectory and compressed sensing with magnitude subtraction. Magn Reson Med 2018;79(2):867–78.

49. Wu H, Block WF, Turski PA, et al. Noncontrast-enhanced three-dimensional (3D) intracranial MR

angiography using pseudocontinuous arterial spin labeling and accelerated 3D radial acquisition. Magn Reson Med 2013;69(3):708–15.

50. Hadizadeh DR, Kukuk GM, Steck DT, et al. Noninvasive evaluation of cerebral arteriovenous malformations by 4D-MRA for preoperative planning and postoperative follow-up in 56 patients: comparison with DSA and intraoperative findings. AJNR Am J Neuroradiol 2012;33(6):1095–101.

51. Xu J, Shi D, Chen C, et al. Noncontrast-enhanced four-dimensional MR angiography for the evaluation of cerebral arteriovenous malformation: a preliminary trial. J Magn Reson Imaging 2011;34(5):1199–205.

52. Cong F, Zhuo Y, Yu S, et al. Noncontrast-enhanced time-resolved 4D dynamic intracranial MR angiography at 7T: a feasibility study. J Magn Reson Imaging 2018;48(1):111–20.

53. Qiao Y, Steinman DA, Qin Q, et al. Intracranial arterial wall imaging using three-dimensional high isotropic resolution black blood MRI at 3.0 Tesla. J Magn Reson Imaging 2011;34(1):22–30.

54. Qiao Y, Zeiler SR, Mirbagheri S, et al. Intracranial plaque enhancement in patients with cerebrovascular events on high-spatial-resolution MR images. Radiology 2014;271(2):534–42.

55. Fan Z, Yang Q, Deng Z, et al. Whole-brain intracranial vessel wall imaging at 3 Tesla using cerebrospinal fluid–attenuated T1-weighted 3 D turbo spin echo. Magn Reson Med 2017;77(3):1142–50.

56. Van Der Kolk A, Zwanenburg J, Denswil N, et al. Imaging the intracranial atherosclerotic vessel wall using 7T MRI: initial comparison with histopathology. AJNR Am J Neuroradiol 2015;36(4):694–701.

57. Cho ZH, Kang CK, Han JY, et al. Observation of the lenticulostriate arteries in the human brain in vivo using 7.0T MR angiography. Stroke 2008;39(5):1604–6.

58. Ma SJ, Sarabi MS, Wang K, et al. Deep Learning segmentation of lenticulostriate arteries on 3D black blood MRI. In. Vol 28. Proceedings of ISMRM 2020;1305.

59. Dury RJ, Falah Y, Gowland PA, et al. Ultra-high-field arterial spin labelling MRI for non-contrast assessment of cortical lesion perfusion in multiple sclerosis. Eur Radiol 2019;29(4):2027–33.

60. Wu W-C, Lin S-C, Wang DJ, et al. Measurement of cerebral white matter perfusion using pseudocontinuous arterial spin labeling 3T magnetic resonance imaging–an experimental and theoretical investigation of feasibility. PLoS One 2013;8(12):e82679.

61. Ma SJ, Jann K, Barisano G, et al. Characterization of lenticulostriate arteries using arterial spin labeling and high-resolution 3D black-blood MRI as an imaging marker in vascular cognitive impairment and dementia. Alzheimer's Dementia 2019;15(7):P1103–4.

62. Balchandani P, Khalighi MM, Hsieh SS, et al. Adiabatic B1 Shimming algorithm for multiple channel transmit at 7T. Proc ISMRM 2011;19:2907.

63. Katscher U, Bornert P, Leussler C, et al. Transmit SENSE. Magn Reson Med 2003;49(1):144–50.

Perivascular Space Imaging at Ultrahigh Field MR Imaging

Giuseppe Barisano, MD[a],*, Meng Law, MD[b], Rachel M. Custer, MS[c],
Arthur W. Toga, PhD[c], Farshid Sepehrband, PhD[c]

KEYWORDS

• Ultrahigh field (UHF) MR imaging • 7 T • Perivascular spaces • Neurovascular imaging

KEY POINTS

• Ultrahigh field (UHF) MR imaging systems have higher signal-to-noise ratio and contrast-to-noise ratio compared with lower field systems, resulting in improved spatial resolution and/or shorter scan times. This allows for visualization of normal and pathologic structures in greater detail.
• UHF MR imaging can be applied to image perivascular spaces (PVS) in vivo, with advantages in the identification and accurate quantification of PVS.
• UHF MR imaging presents some technical challenges and limitations relating to safety issues that must be considered.

INTRODUCTION

Perivascular spaces (PVS), also known as Virchow-Robin spaces, are fluid-filled spaces surrounding arterioles, venules, and capillaries in the brain parenchyma.[1] They were originally identified and described in the nineteenth century,[2] but their function is still not well understood.[3] Recent evidence indicates that PVS constitute a major component of the brain clearance system, playing a critical role in the maintenance of brain health.[3] In fact, PVS are involved in the drainage of the cerebrospinal fluid (CSF) from the subarachnoid space and interstitial fluid from the extracellular space, contributing to the elimination of metabolic waste products from the brain.[4,5]

PVS can be visualized in vivo using MR imaging, where they appear as structures following the course of the blood vessels (arteries and veins) penetrating the cerebral parenchyma, with signal intensity similar to the CSF (ie, dark on T1-weighted and bright on T2-weighted images) and with shape varying from linear to punctate, depending on whether the enclosed blood vessel is oriented parallel or perpendicular to the image acquisition plane, respectively. It should also be noted that PVS and enclosed blood vessels currently cannot be easily differentiated on MR imaging and therefore appear as a unique tubular structure.

Although the clinical application of MR imaging dates back to the 1980s, only in the past 2 decades clinicians and researchers have started to visualize and analyze cerebral PVS on MR imaging (particularly at higher resolution and field strength). Such analysis of morphologic features and alterations of the PVS associated with pathologic conditions has been substantially facilitated by improvements to imaging sequences and postprocessing techniques, which allow for enhancement of image quality and resolution. More recently, the use of ultrahigh field (UHF) MR imaging systems (≥7 T)

[a] Neuroscience Graduate Program, University of Southern California, 2025 Zonal Ave, Los Angeles, CA 90033, USA; [b] Department of Neuroscience, Central Clinical School, Monash University, The Alfred Health, Level 6, 99 Commercial Road, Melbourne, Victoria 3004, Australia; [c] Laboratory of Neuro Imaging, Stevens Neuroimaging and Informatics Institute, Keck School of Medicine, University of Southern California, 2025 Zonal Ave, Los Angeles, CA 90033, USA
* Corresponding author.
E-mail address: giuseppe.barisano@loni.usc.edu

Magn Reson Imaging Clin N Am 29 (2021) 67–75
https://doi.org/10.1016/j.mric.2020.09.005
1064-9689/21/© 2020 Elsevier Inc. All rights reserved.

have enabled even greater increases in spatial resolution due to the higher signal-to-noise ratios (SNR), resulting in significantly enhanced evaluation and visualization of PVS.

Here the authors describe sequences and postprocessing techniques for PVS imaging, the main limitations of UHF MR imaging for PVS, and the latest findings regarding PVS imaged at 7 T MR imaging.

NEUROIMAGING TECHNIQUES FOR PERIVASCULAR SPACES ANALYSIS

Previous MR imaging studies in humans have demonstrated that a higher number of visible PVS have been associated with several clinical conditions, including neuropsychiatric and sleep disorders,[6–10] multiple sclerosis,[11,12] mild traumatic brain injury,[13,14] Parkinson disease,[15] post-traumatic epilepsy,[14] myotonic dystrophy,[16] systemic lupus erythematosus,[17] cerebral small vessel disease,[18–22] and cerebral amyloid-β pathologies, such as Alzheimer disease (AD) and cerebral amyloid angiopathy.[23–28] These findings suggest that alterations of PVS indicate underlying cerebral pathology, and as a result, increasing attention has been dedicated to the in vivo analysis of PVS using MR imaging.

The PVS visible on MR imaging are filled with a CSF-like fluid, that is, a fluid with a low level of proteins and macromolecules, causing PVS to predominantly exhibit T2 properties on MR imaging, appearing bright on T2-weighted images with long repetition time and echo time. In fact, T2-weighted image is currently considered the most appropriate sequence to visualize PVS because the contrast PVS white matter is higher when compared with the same contrast on T1-weighted images. Turbo spin echo (TSE) sequences, such as 3D TSE-based SPACE (Sampling Perfection with Application optimized Contrasts by using different flip angle Evolutions—Siemens), or 3-dimensional fast spin echo (FSE) equivalents such as 3D T2 CUBE (GE), 3D T2 VISTA (Volume ISotropic Turbo spin echo Acquisition—Phillips), or 3D MVOX (MultiVOXel—Canon), have been shown to be particularly suitable for analyzing PVS on MR imaging, especially at UHF,[29–32] offering isotropic or almost isotropic spatial resolution (up to 0.4 mm³) and near whole-brain coverage with a scan time of approximately 10 minutes.[33]

Although on conventional 1.5 T MR imaging the visibility of PVS is mostly limited to those that are dilated or tumefactive, recent advancements in sequence development and the more widespread use of high-field (3 T) and UHF MR imaging enable improved visualization of PVS in general, not only enlarged PVS, but also normal, physiologic, or nondilated PVS.

At 7 T, for example, the higher SNR (more than double that achievable with a 3 T MR imaging system) allows for an increase in spatial resolution from the reduction of voxel size. This has provided a significantly improved visualization of PVS on MR imaging, especially for smaller PVS (<1 mm), and has increased the ability to study their morphologic features and distribution at the mesoscale (Fig. 1).

In addition to methods for improving image acquisition, researchers have also investigated new postprocessing approaches to enhance the visibility of PVS on MR imaging and consequently, to obtain more accurate quantitation of PVS. Various approaches for enhancing visualization of PVS have been reported in the past few years. For example, Uchiyama and colleagues[34] were able to enhance the signal intensity of PVS and lacunar infarcts on T2-weighted images at 1.5 T by applying the morphologic "white" top-hat transformation. More recently, the Haar transform of nonlocal cubes was used to enhance the signal of PVS on T2-weighted images acquired at 7 T MR imaging followed by a block-matching 4-dimensional filtering to suppress the noise.[35] Another recent work at 7 T MR imaging described the employment of Densely Connected Deep Convolutional Neural Networks to enhance the PVS signal and to suppress the noise without the need for heuristic parameter tuning, which is required for other techniques previously described.[36] Finally, Sepehrband and colleagues[37] have shown that an enhanced PVS contrast image can be obtained by dividing denoised T1-weighted and T2-weighted images (Fig. 2). This technique was developed using 3 T MR imaging scans but can potentially be applied to images acquired at 7 T as well.

The ultimate goal of these techniques is to facilitate the visual analysis, segmentation, and quantitation of PVS on MR imaging.

Because pathologic changes to PVS are expected to initiate in submillimeter scales,[38] the use of UHF MR imaging and/or techniques to enhance the PVS visibility for quantitation is fundamental not only for the analysis of physiologic nondilated PVS but also to identify the early and more subtle pathologic changes occurring in PVS. The identification of these features may be found to play a critical role in the diagnosis of various diseases and can provide essential insights into the physiology and pathophysiology of the PVS, which will be important for the investigation and development of new potential therapeutic strategies for

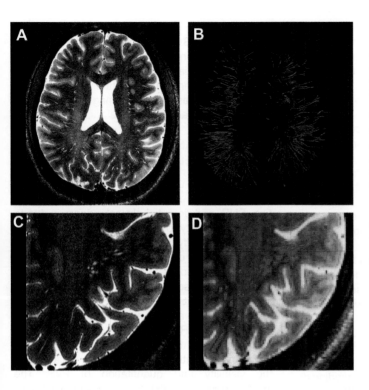

Fig. 1. Visualization and measures of PVS on MR imaging depend on the image resolution. (*A*) Axial T2-weighted 3D SPACE image at 7T from a healthy 26-year-old male volunteer acquired at 0.32 × 0.32 × 0.4 mm resolution (interpolated to 0.16 × 0.16 × 0.4 mm) with the following parameters: GRAPPA = 3, TR/TE = 2320/299 ms, flip angle = 120, 2 averages. Scan time: 24 minutes. (*B*) Manual segmentation of the PVS across a subportion (8 cm slab) of the white matter. (*C, D*) Comparison of PVS segmentation at high resolution (C: 0.16 × 0.16 × 0.4 mm) and moderate resolution (D: 0.6 mm³) on 7T MR imaging. PVS characteristics and morphologic features were overestimated when 0.6 mm³ resolution image was used, especially for the smaller PVSs. The image in D has been acquired from the same volunteer using the following parameters: GRAPPA = 3, TR/TE = 2140/221 ms. Scan time: 11 minutes. GRAPPA, generalized autocalibrating partially parallel acquisitions; TR/TE, repetition time/echo time.

diseases associated with alterations in cerebral blood flow, CSF/lymphatic drainage, and resultant changes in the PVS.

In addition to structural MR imaging, PVS can also be studied with diffusion-weighted MR (dMR) imaging. Recent evidence shows that PVS significantly and systematically influences dMR imaging metrics when a dMR imaging acquisition is performed with multiple b-values (multishell dMR imaging), which allows for differentiation of the PVS fluid component from the white matter signal.[37] Diffusion MR imaging enables the study of properties of the fluid within the PVS along with the PVS microstructural changes themselves, with significant implications in terms of pathophysiology. For example, it has been demonstrated that the PVS fluid signal can predict pathologic increases in mean diffusivity found in early cognitive decline.[38] At UHF, dMR imaging benefits from the higher spatial resolution and reduction of partial

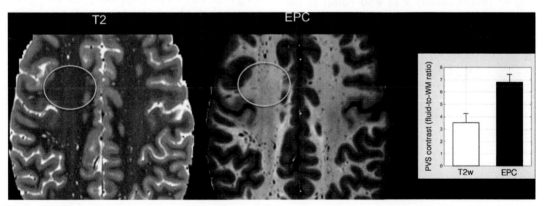

Fig. 2. The PVS visibility is enhanced on enhanced PVS contrast (EPC) compared with T2-weighted images. Example showing a T2-weighted image at 3 T from a healthy young volunteer acquired at 0.7 mm³ resolution and the corresponding EPC image. The visibility of PVS is improved on EPC, especially in areas with small PVS and/or multiple PVS close to each other. In fact, the contrast PVS/white matter was on average higher on EPC compared with T2-weighted images.

volume effects, resulting in a more accurate separation of multiple parenchymal compartments, including fiber bundles in white matter and PVS.[39–42] PVS have been shown to have significant contributions to diffusion signal.[39,40] Unlike the highly hindered interstitial fluid of the white matter, water molecules of PVS fluid can diffuse relatively unbounded when acquiring conventional dMR imaging data. Therefore, even a small *volume fraction* of the PVS fluid in the imaged voxel has a large signal contribution (high *signal fraction*). With high-resolution dMR imaging at UHF, the contribution of PVS becomes more evident in comparison with the lower field MR imaging. Given the high diffusivity of PVS, its signal contribution is largest at low b-values (<1000 s/mm^2).

To assess the contribution of PVS to diffusion signal at UHF, we conducted a multishell dMR imaging experiment and compared diffusion signal in the same anatomic regions with and without PVS presence. A 50-minute scan was conducted to acquire dMR imaging volumes at the following b-values: 0, 200, 400, 600, 800 s/mm^2 with fixed echo time of 65 ms, TR of 4400 ms, and isotropic resolution of 1.3 mm^3. Thirty gradient-encoding directions per shell were acquired in both anterior-posterior and posterior-anterior phase encoding directions. Regions of the putamen of the basal ganglia with high vascular density were manually segmented (**Fig. 3**A). Basal ganglia were chosen because this region is known to have high vascular and PVS presence, allowing for comparison of PVS fluid with perfusion-related diffusion changes, also known as intravoxel incoherent motion.[43] Experimental data showed that PVS fluid explains fast diffusion signal decay at low b-values (200–800 s/mm^2). The region with high PVS exhibits a faster signal decay (see **Fig. 3**B,C). As expected, a higher proton density was also noted in the

high PVS region (higher S_0 signal). These results suggest that PVS fluid has a different diffusion profile in comparison with the rest of the extracellular fluid (ie, interstitial fluid) and therefore should be modeled accordingly for quantitative techniques.

The advantages of 7 T MR imaging for PVS imaging are summarized in **Table 1**.

LIMITATIONS AND DISADVANTAGES OF ULTRAHIGH FIELD MR IMAGING

Even though the use of UHF MR imaging can provide remarkable improvements in spatial resolution, SNR, and potential clinical outcomes due to its superior ability to depict small anatomic structures and identify more subtle pathology,[41,44,45] there are several challenges and limitations related to UHF that need to be taken into account. Here the authors describe the issues they consider important for PVS imaging at UHF.

Because PVS appear as relatively small structures in brain MR imaging scans and are distributed throughout the white matter, it is crucial to have images without artifacts that could affect the visibility and quantitation of PVS. The increased SNR of UHF MR imaging could certainly reduce the scan time, which is one critical factor influencing the likelihood of acquiring images with motion artifact. However, increased spatial resolution usually goes along with increased sensitivity to motion, potentially resulting in a higher incidence of artifacts caused by movement of the individual being scanned, such as blurring, ringing, and ghosting.[46] To a lesser extent, these artifacts can also be determined by physiologic involuntary and/or spontaneous movements, including heartbeat, respiration, and minor/subtle head movements.[47] This issue may be significantly mitigated and often completely solved by the employment of motion correction procedures.

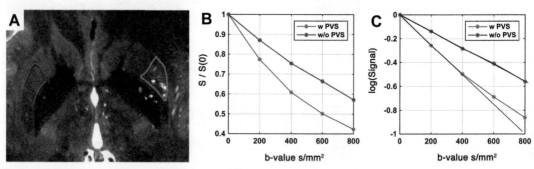

Fig. 3. PVS fluid has significant contribution to diffusion signal at low b-value. (*A*) Both the studied regions have high vascular presence (lenticulostriate arteries penetrate into the putamen). Two regions of interest with low PVS (*red*) and high PVS (*blue*) presence were manually delineated. (*B, C*) Normalized diffusion signal and the log form in these regions are shown. Note that the region with high PVS presence decays faster and shows a biexponential profile.

Table 1
Advantages of 7T MR imaging for perivascular spaces imaging

PVS Feature	7 T Advantage
Visibility	Improved visibility at 7 T
Count	More PVS can be counted at 7 T (smaller PVS can be detected)
Volume	Higher accuracy at 7 T (partial volume effect at lower field results in overestimation of the PVS volume)
Caliber	Higher accuracy at 7 T (partial volume effect at lower field results in overestimation of the PVS caliber)
Solidity	Higher accuracy at 7 T (PVS can be mapped in more depth into the parenchyma, allowing the measurement of solidity)
Diffusion	PVS affect diffusion signal, especially at low b-value (<1000 s/mm^2).

For example, prospective motion correction systems using a camera and a moiré phase tracking marker allow identification of head movements to minute levels to dynamically adjust the imaging protocol in real time.[48,49] In addition, postacquisition procedures and deep learning methods can be used to perform a retrospective and prospective correction of involuntary microscopic head movement.[50] Both types of motion correction techniques will lead to improved image quality under UHF MR imaging.[51,52]

As reported earlier, high contrast and SNR constitute 2 key elements for the optimal and accurate visualization of PVS on MR imaging. Although UHF provides higher SNR than MR imaging systems at lower field strength, it is important to consider that the Larmor frequency for protons in the human head increases as well, and therefore the transmit radiofrequency (RF) magnetic field (B$_1$) results in inhomogeneity because the RF wavelength of B$_1$ becomes smaller than anatomic structures in the main magnetic field.[53] The increase in B$_1$ inhomogeneity alters the contrast-to-noise ratio and flip angles across the field of view, resulting in a progressive decrease of SNR from the central part of brain to the periphery.[41] B$_1$ inhomogeneity is particularly problematic for PVS imaging because it especially affects spin echo–based sequences, including T2-weighted, due to magnetization refocusing.[54–58] Moreover, because the course of PVS in the white matter tends to be centripetal, extending from the subcortical white matter toward the lateral ventricles, the loss of SNR in the periphery may significantly influence the ability to detect the subcortical portion of PVS. The 2 most common solutions to try to alleviate the effects related to B$_1$ inhomogeneities are the following: the employment of transmit and receive RF parallel coil arrays (parallel transmit/receive), which can model the RF pulse sequences on each channel enhancing the

B$_1$ homogeneity,[59] and the use of adiabatic RF pulses, which improves the outer volume suppression by controlling and adjusting the frequency and amplitude of B$_1$ above the adiabatic threshold.[60]

The next 2 challenges are related to the safety of the subjects undergoing the MR imaging scan at UHF. Specific absorption rate (SAR) is the amount of RF energy absorbed by the human body during the scan, followed by an increase in temperature. SAR not only exhibits approximately a quadratic growth with the magnetic field but is also significantly increased by the use of sequences with large and/or very rapid RF pulses, including TSE, which is commonly used for PVS imaging. In order to avoid an excessively high SAR, parallel imaging techniques, such as generalized autocalibrating partially parallel acquisitions, can be used; moreover, reducing flip angles and increasing TR may be convenient to lower SAR, although it may lead to longer acquisition times. It should be noted that, for safety purposes, MR imaging scanners generally prevent initiation of the acquisition of images with sequences where estimated SAR is close or above the limits set by the Food and Drug Administration (for brain MR imaging: 38°C or 3.2 W/kg averaged overhead mass).

Finally, all individuals entering an MR environment need to be screened for biomedical implants and devices. This is particularly critical at UHF, as presently only a limited number of implants have been tested and approved for 7 T MR imaging scanners, which precludes the use of UHF MR imaging in subjects with untested implants.[61–64] Recently, safety guidelines for health care professionals have been proposed in order to ensure safety in research subjects or patients with metallic implants referred for 7 T scans, including those with untested implants.[65] In general, an accurate scrutiny of the potential risk versus benefit of the MR imaging examination for each individual as well as an analysis of the material, anatomic location, and type of implant are the most important aspects to consider when deciding whether or not to proceed with the scan.[65]

LATEST RESEARCH IN PERIVASCULAR SPACES AT ULTRAHIGH FIELD MR IMAGING

In the past few years, several groups used 7 T MR imaging systems to investigate PVS, both under physiologic conditions and in pathology. The first study of PVS at 7 T reported the feasibility of imaging and quantification of PVS at UHF and confirmed, in a small sample size, that PVS density in patients with AD was significantly higher compared with age-matched healthy controls,[31] as previously demonstrated at lower field strength.[23–28] Another recent paper investigated whether PVS may represent a new biomarker for epilepsy.[29] The investigators manually counted PVS using axial T2-weighted TSE sequences acquired in 21 patients with focal epilepsy and 17 healthy volunteers. They found that patients with epilepsy presented a more asymmetric distribution of PVS; in 72% of cases, the region of maximum asymmetry matched with the suspected seizure onset zone, with less PVS visible in that area compared with the contralateral side.[29] The relationship between PVS asymmetry and epilepsy was interpreted as an effect of the disease on cerebral structures, possibly determined by the disrupted macrophage activity in the seizure onset zone.[29]

The advancements in PVS analysis on MR imaging have allowed for further study of PVS not only in disease but also in physiologic states. To date, the normal amount and distribution of PVS in healthy human brains have not been fully described nor understood, and therefore the ability to confidently define the pathogenic alterations in PVS, especially in subclinical stages of diseases, is hindered. Recently, 2 groups analyzed PVS in healthy volunteers using 7 T MR imaging. Bouvy and colleagues[32] showed that PVS were spatially correlated with lenticulostriate arteries in the basal ganglia and with perforating arteries in the centrum semiovale but not with veins. Moreover, a higher number of PVS was found in older adults (n = 5, age: 51–72 years) compared with younger people (n = 5, age: 19–27 years), but no differences in PVS diameter were reported.[32] Zong and colleagues[33] described the PVS morphology and distribution in the basal ganglia, thalamus, midbrain, and white matter of 45 healthy subjects (age: 21–55 yeas) scanned at 7 T. They found that PVS count and volume fraction significantly increased with age in basal ganglia and

presented high intersubject variability as well as a significant spatial heterogeneity not solely explained by B_1 inhomogeneities.[33] They also showed that carbogen breathing significantly increased the PVS volume fraction in basal ganglia and white matter,[33] which suggests a link between vasodilation and apparent PVS volume on MR imaging. Further studies with larger sample size will be required to better understand the morphologic features of PVS in normal conditions and which factors affect the physiologic appearance of PVS on MR imaging.

SUMMARY

Current results show that imaging PVS at UHF is feasible and offers the possibility of accurately identifying and quantitation of the PVS, including those smaller in size (<1 mm), which are usually not visible on conventional lower field MR imaging scans. This may be particularly helpful in analyzing the normal PVS and the early pathologic alterations of PVS. More studies, both in clinical and research settings, are required to investigate the advantages of UHF for in vivo PVS analysis, and this will allow further investigation into the physiologic function of PVS in terms of cerebrospinal-interstitial fluid exchange, lymphatic and brain clearance system, as well as their role as a diagnostic biomarker for some neurologic diseases. Moreover, further efforts are needed to solve the existing limitations of imaging at UHF, including both those related to sequence optimization and hardware development and those concerning SAR limitations and the safety of subjects and patients. Nonetheless, the more widespread application of UHF MR imaging systems is expected to result in novel scientific discoveries and more opportunities to use 7 T MR imaging scanners as diagnostic tools in clinics, with subsequent anticipated improvement of the clinical outcomes of patients.

ACKNOWLEDGMENTS

Research reported in this publication was supported by the National Institute of Mental Health of the National Institutes of Health under Award Number RF1MH123223. The content is solely the responsibility of the authors and does not necessarily represent the official views of the National Institutes of Health.

DISCLOSURE

The authors have nothing to disclose.

REFERENCES

1. Zhang ET, Inman CB, Weller RO. Interrelationships of the pia mater and the perivascular (Virchow-Robin) spaces in the human cerebrum. J Anat 1990;170:111.

2. Woollam DH, Millen JW. The perivascular spaces of the mammalian central nervous system and their relation to the perineuronal and subarachnoid spaces. J Anat 1955;89(2):193–200.

3. Wardlaw JM, Benveniste H, Nedergaard M, et al. Perivascular spaces in the brain: anatomy, physiology, and contributions to pathology of brain diseases. Nat Res 2020;16:137–53.

4. Rasmussen MK, Mestre H, Nedergaard M. The glymphatic pathway in neurological disorders. Lancet Neurol 2018;17(11):1016–24.

5. Tarasoff-Conway JM, Carare RO, Osorio RS, et al. Clearance systems in the brain—implications for Alzheimer disease. Nat Rev Neurol 2015;11(8):457.

6. MacLullich AMJ, Wardlaw JM, Ferguson KJ, et al. Enlarged perivascular spaces are associated with cognitive function in healthy elderly men. J Neurol Neurosurg Psychiatry 2004;75(11):1519–23.

7. Taber KH, Shaw JB, Loveland KA, et al. Accentuated Virchow-Robin spaces in the centrum semiovale in children with Autistic disorder. J Comput Assist Tomogr 2004;28(2):263–8.

8. Rollins NK, Deline C, Morriss MC. Prevalence and clinical significance of dilated Virchow-Robin spaces in childhood. Radiology 1993;189:53–7.

9. Patankar TF, Baldwin R, Mitra D, et al. Virchow-Robin space dilatation may predict resistance to antidepressant monotherapy in elderly patients with depression. J Affect Disord 2007;97(1–3):265–70.

10. Berezuk C, Ramirez J, Gao F, et al. Virchow-Robin spaces: correlations with polysomnography-derived sleep parameters. Sleep 2015;38(6):853–8.

11. Achiron A, Faibel M. Sandlike appearance of Virchow-Robin spaces in early multiple sclerosis: a novel neuroradiologic marker. Am J Neuroradiol 2002;23(3):376–80.

12. Wuerfel J, Haertle M, Waiczies H, et al. Perivascular spaces–MRI marker of inflammatory activity in the brain? Brain 2008;131(9):2332–40.

13. Inglese M, Bomsztyk E, Gonen O, et al. Dilated perivascular spaces: hallmarks of mild traumatic brain injury. Am J Neuroradiol 2005;26(4).

14. Duncan D, Barisano G, Cabeen R, et al. Analytic tools for post-traumatic epileptogenesis biomarker search in multimodal dataset of an animal model and human patients. Front Neuroinform 2018;12:86.

15. Laitinen LV, Chudy D, Tengvar M, et al. Dilated perivascular spaces in the putamen and pallidum in patients with Parkinson's disease scheduled for pallidotomy: a comparison between MRI findings and clinical symptoms and signs. Mov Disord 2000;15(6):1139–44.

16. Di Costanzo A, Di Salle F, Santoro L, et al. Dilated Virchow-Robin spaces in myotonic dystrophy: frequency, extent and significance. Eur Neurol 2001; 46(3):131–9.

17. Miyata M, Kakeda S, Iwata S, et al. Enlarged perivascular spaces are associated with the disease activity in systemic lupus erythematosus. Sci Rep 2017;7(1):1–10.

18. Potter GM, Doubal FN, Jackson CA, et al. Enlarged perivascular spaces and cerebral small vessel disease. Int J Stroke 2015;10(3):376–81.

19. Rouhl RPW, Van Oostenbrugge RJ, Knottnerus ILH, et al. Virchow-Robin spaces relate to cerebral small vessel disease severity. J Neurol 2008;255(5): 692–6.

20. Ohba H, Pearce L, Potter G, et al. Enlarged perivascular spaces in lacunar stroke patients. The secondary prevention of small subcortical stroked (SPS3) trial. Stroke 2012;43:A151.

21. Doubal FN, MacLullich AMJ, Ferguson KJ, et al. Enlarged perivascular spaces on MRI are a feature of cerebral small vessel disease. Stroke 2010; 41(3):450–4.

22. Wardlaw JM, Smith EE, Biessels GJ, et al. Neuroimaging standards for research into small vessel disease and its contribution to ageing and neurodegeneration. Lancet Neurol 2013;12(8): 822–38.

23. Charidimou A, Jaunmuktane Z, Baron J-C, et al. White matter perivascular spaces: an MRI marker in pathology-proven cerebral amyloid angiopathy? Neurology 2014;82(1):57–62.

24. Martinez-Ramirez S, Pontes-Neto OM, Dumas AP, et al. Topography of dilated perivascular spaces in subjects from a memory clinic cohort. Neurology 2013;80(17):1551–6.

25. Rohor AE, Kuo Y M, Esh C, et al. Cortical and leptomeningeal cerebrovascular amyloid and white matter pathology in Alzheimer's disease. Mol Med 2003;9(3–4):112–22.

26. Ramirez J, Berezuk C, McNeely AA, et al. Visible Virchow-Robin spaces on magnetic resonance imaging of Alzheimer's disease patients and normal elderly from the Sunnybrook dementia study. J Alzheimer's Dis 2015;43(2):415–24.

27. Hansen TP, Cain J, Thomas O, et al. Dilated perivascular spaces in the Basal Ganglia are a biomarker of small-vessel disease in a very elderly population with dementia. AJNR Am J Neuroradiol 2015;36(5): 893–8.

28. Chen W, Song X, Zhang Y. Assessment of the virchow-robin spaces in Alzheimer disease, mild cognitive impairment, and normal aging, using high-field MR imaging. Am J Neuroradiol 2011; 32(8):1490–5.

29. Feldman RE, Rutland JW, Fields MC, et al. Quantification of perivascular spaces at 7T: a potential MRI biomarker for epilepsy. Seizure 2018;54:11–8.

30. Zong X, Park SH, Shen D, et al. Visualization of perivascular spaces in the human brain at 7T: sequence optimization and morphology characterization. Neuroimage 2016;125:895–902.

31. Cai K, Wain R, Das S, et al. The feasibility of quantitative MRI of perivascular spaces at 7T. J Neurosci Methods 2015;269:151–6.

32. Bouvy WH, Biessels GJ, Kuijf HJ, et al. Visualization of perivascular spaces and perforating arteries with 7 T magnetic resonance imaging. Invest Radiol 2014;49(5):307–13.

33. Zong X, Lian C, Jimenez J, et al. Morphology of perivascular spaces and enclosed blood vessels in young to middle-aged healthy adults at 7T: dependences on age, brain region, and breathing gas. Neuroimage 2020;218:116978.

34. Uchiyama Y, Kunieda T, Asano T, et al. Computer-aided diagnosis scheme for classification of lacunar infarcts and enlarged Virchow-Robin spaces in brain MR images. In: Proceedings of the 30th Annual International Conference of the IEEE Engineering in Medicine and Biology Society, EMBS'08 - "Personalized healthcare through Technology." Vol 2008. Conf Proc IEEE Eng Med Biol Soc. Vancouver, BC, Canada, August 20–24, 2008. doi:10.1109/iembs.2008.4650064.

35. Hou Y, Park SH, Wang Q, et al. Enhancement of perivascular spaces in 7 T MR image using Haar transform of non-local cubes and block-matching filtering. Sci Rep 2017;7(1):8569.

36. Jung E, Chikontwe P, Zong X, et al. Enhancement of perivascular spaces using densely connected deep convolutional neural network. IEEE Access 2019;7: 18382–91.

37. Sepehrband F, Barisano G, Sheikh-Bahaei N, et al. Image processing approaches to enhance perivascular space visibility and quantification using MRI. Sci Rep 2019;9:12351.

38. Shi Y, Wardlaw JM. Update on cerebral small vessel disease: a dynamic whole-brain disease. Stroke and Vascular Neurology 2016;1:83–92.

39. Sepehrband F, Cabeen RP, Choupan J, et al. Perivascular space fluid contributes to diffusion tensor imaging changes in white matter. Neuroimage 2019;197:243–54.

40. Sepehrband F, Cabeen RP, Barisano G, et al. Non-parenchymal fluid is the source of increased mean diffusivity in preclinical Alzheimer's disease. Alzheimer Dement (Amst) 2019;11:348–54.

41. Barisano G, Sepehrband F, Ma S, et al. Clinical 7 T MRI: Are we there yet? A review about magnetic resonance imaging at ultra-high field. Br J Radiol 2018;91:20180492.

42. Sepehrband F, O'Brien K, Barth M. A time-efficient acquisition protocol for multipurpose diffusion-weighted microstructural imaging at 7 Tesla. Magn Reson Med 2017;78(6):2170–84.

43. Le Bihan D. IVIM method measures diffusion and perfusion. Diagn Imaging (San Franc) 1990;12(6): 133–6.

44. Balchandani P, Naidich TP. Ultra-high-field MR neuroimaging. Am J Neuroradiol 2015;36(7):1204–15.

45. Trattnig S, Springer E, Bogner W, et al. Key clinical benefits of neuroimaging at 7 T. Neuroimage 2016. https://doi.org/10.1016/J.NEUROIMAGE.2016.11. 031.

46. Zaitsev M, Maclaren J, Herbst M. Motion artifacts in MRI: A complex problem with many partial solutions. J Magn Reson Imaging 2015;42(4):887–901.

47. Herbst M, MacLaren J, Lovell-Smith C, et al. Reproduction of motion artifacts for performance analysis of prospective motion correction in MRI. Magn Reson Med 2014;71(1):182–90.

48. Schulz J, Siegert T, Reimer E, et al. An embedded optical tracking system for motion-corrected magnetic resonance imaging at 7T. MAGMA 2012; 25(6):443–53.

49. Maclaren J, Armstrong BSR, Barrows RT, et al. Measurement and correction of microscopic head motion during magnetic resonance imaging of the brain. PLoS One 2012;7(11).

50. Gallichan D, Marques JP, Gruetter R. Retrospective correction of involuntary microscopic head movement using highly accelerated fat image navigators (3D FatNavs) at 7T. Magn Reson Med 2016;75(3): 1030–9.

51. Stucht D, Danishad KA, Schulze P, et al. Highest resolution in vivo human brain MRI using prospective motion correction. PLoS One 2015;10(7):1–17.

52. Federau C, Gallichan D. Motion-correction enabled ultra-high resolution in-vivo 7T-MRI of the brain. PLoS One 2016;11(5).

53. Ibrahim TS, Lee R, Baertlein BA, et al. Effect of RF coil excitation on field inhomogeneity at ultra high fields: A field optimized TEM resonatior. Magn Reson Imaging 2001;19(10):1339–47.

54. Poon CS, Henkelman RM. Practical T2 quantitation for clinical applications. J Magn Reson Imaging 1992;2(5):541–53.

55. Norris DG, Koopmans PJ, Boyacioğlu R, et al. Power independent of number of slices (PINS) radiofrequency pulses for low-power simultaneous multislice excitation. Magn Reson Med 2011;66(5): 1234–40.

56. Majumdar S, Orphanoudakis SC, Gmitro A, et al. Errors in the measurements of T2 using multiple-echo MRI techniques. I. Effects of radiofrequency pulse imperfections. Magn Reson Med 1986;3(3): 397–417.

57. Vargas MI, Martelli P, Xin L, et al. Clinical neuroimaging using 7 T MRI: challenges and prospects. J Neuroimaging 2018;28(1):5–13.

58. Kraff O, Quick HH. 7T: Physics, safety, and potential clinical applications. J Magn Reson Imaging 2017; 46(6):1573–89.

59. Zhu Y. Parallel Excitation with an Array of Transmit Coils. Magn Reson Med 2004;51(4):775–84.

60. Tannús A, Garwood M. Adiabatic pulses. NMR Biomed 1997;10(8):423–34.

61. Sammet CL, Yang X, Wassenaar PA, et al. RF-related heating assessment of extracranial neurosurgical implants at 7T. Magn Reson Imaging 2013; 31(6):1029–34.

62. Feng DX, McCauley JP, Morgan-Curtis FK, et al. Evaluation of 39 medical implants at 7.0T. Br J Radiol 2015;88(1056):1–10.

63. Dula AN, Virostko J, Shellock FG. Assessment of MRI issues at 7 T for 28 implants and other objects. Am J Roentgenol 2014;202(2):401–5.

64. Shellock FG. Reference manual for magnetic resonance safety, implants, and devices: 2018 edition. Los Angeles (CA): Biomedical Research Publishing Group; 2018.

65. Barisano G, Culo B, Shellock FG, et al. 7-Tesla MRI of the brain in a research subject with bilateral, total knee replacement implants: case report and proposed safety guidelines. Magn Reson Imaging 2019;57:313–6.

Dynamic Glucose-Enhanced MR Imaging

Daniel Paech, MD, MS[a],*, Alexander Radbruch, MD, JD[b]

KEYWORDS

- Glucose-enhanced MR imaging • Chemical exchange saturation transfer (CEST)
- Chemical exchange-sensitive spin-lock (CESL) • MR biomarkers • GlucoCEST • GlucoCESL

KEY POINTS

- Dynamic glucose-enhanced (DGE) MR imaging is a novel MR contrast that uses natural glucose solution as biodegradable contrast agent.
- DGE MR imaging particularly profits from ultrahigh field strength (7T and higher) due to increased signal-to-noise ratio.
- DGE MR imaging may aid tumor detection and characterization due to high glucose demand of cancer cells.

INTRODUCTION

Contrast agents have become an integral part of daily clinical imaging. In MR imaging, the most widely used contrast agent contains the metal gadolinium that is chelated to avoid the potential toxic effects of gadolinium. Generally, gadolinium-based contrast agents (GBCA) have an excellent safety profile and have been applied worldwide more than 500 million times. However, GBCAs have garnered some discussion in recent years, as several studies reported traces of gadolinium in the brain following serial injections of GBCAs.[1-7] The effect has been primarily seen with the so-called linear GBCAs, and less gadolinium has been found when the more stable macrocyclic GBCAs were administered. Importantly, no clinical correlates or findings of these gadolinium depositions have been shown. However, common sense dictates that it is preferable to avoid any metal accumulation in the patient. Thus various imaging techniques have been proposed to reduce or substitute gadolinium administration. Obviously, contrast agents that naturally appear in the human body would be preferable substitutes. Especially, the natural D-glucose could be a promising candidate when adequate MR imaging techniques are used. In the following the authors provide an overview of the current state of the art technique for the imaging of D-glucose.

MR IMAGING WITH GLUCOSE AS A CONTRAST MEDIUM IN VIVO

Direct detection of glucose using MR imaging or MR spectroscopy has limited spatial resolution due to the very low in vivo glucose concentration.

Chemical exchange (CE)-sensitive MR imaging represents a novel technique enabling the detection of low-concentration metabolites and proteins in vivo with high spatial and temporal resolution. CE-sensitive MR imaging approaches, such as CE saturation transfer (CEST) or CE-sensitive spin-lock (CESL), are based on the spontaneous exchange between solute-bound protons and protons of free bulk water yielding signal amplification of several orders of magnitude.[8] In living tissue, multiple different endogenous CE signals from

Conflict of interest: The authors declare no conflict of interest.

Funding: D. Paech is funded by the DFG (German Research Foundation).

[a] Division of Radiology, German Cancer Research Center (DKFZ), Im Neuenheimer Feld 280, Heidelberg 69120, Germany; [b] Clinic for Diagnostic and Interventional Neuroradiology, Venusberg Campus 1, Bonn 53127, Germany

* Corresponding author.

E-mail address: d.paech@dkfz.de

Magn Reson Imaging Clin N Am 29 (2021) 77–81

https://doi.org/10.1016/j.mric.2020.09.009

proteins,[9–11] creatine,[12,13] and glutamate[14,15] as well as exogenously administered substances such as natural glucose[8,16–18] can be observed (**Fig. 1**).

The feasibility of measuring the uptake of exogenously administered glucose during an MR imaging experiment was initially demonstrated in preclinical studies using both CEST [17,19–22] and CESL [23–25] approaches at ultrahigh field strength.

Generally, a DGE MR imaging experiment can be subdivided into 3 phases:

1. "Baseline phase:" the baseline signal is acquired over a defined period (eg, a few minutes) before glucose administration.
2. "Injection phase:" glucose is administered intravenously (eg, 140 mM and 0.2 mL in animals[17]; eg, 100 mL 20% D-glucose in humans[16]) during continuous data acquisition with high temporal resolution.
3. "Decay phase:" from a technical point of view, the "decay phase" is a continuation of the second phase with continuous data acquisition and slow signal decay.

The total measurement duration mainly depends on the length of the third phase (usually between 20 and 40 minutes; however, further shortening is principally feasible). The DGE MR imaging contrast is given by the (relative) signal intensity difference between S(t), the signal intensity at a time point t, and a reference signal obtained from the baseline. DGE MR imaging contrast are prone to motion-induced artifacts because DGE image series consist of data acquired before, during, and after glucose injection.[26] Therefore, motion correction approaches have recently been developed in order to reduce motion-induced artifacts and to increase methodical robustness of DGE MR imaging.[27]

First results in patients with glioma were reported by Xu and colleagues[18] using CEST MR imaging and by Schuenke and colleagues and Paech and colleagues using an adiabatically prepared CESL technique[8,16,28] (**Fig. 2**).

Tumors of patients with glioblastoma and disrupted blood-brain barrier (BBB) showed increased glucose concentrations following intravenous administration that partially overlapped with corresponding conventional gadolinium-enhanced T1-weighted images[8,18,28] and relative cerebral blood volume maps.[16] Increased glucose concentrations were also reported in areas beyond the disrupted BBB.[16,28]

In healthy volunteers, increased glucose concentrations were reported in cerebral vessels and vascular structures (eg, choroid plexus) and in gray matter tissue compared with white matter.[16,18,29] These results are most likely due to increased glucose concentrations in the vascular compartment (perfusion) following intravenous glucose administration. The underlying signal origin is discussed more detail in the following paragraph.

SIGNAL ORIGIN OF DYNAMIC GLUCOSE-ENHANCED MR IMAGING IN HUMANS

In contrast to GBCA, which are confined to the intravascular space and the extracellular extravascular space (EES), glucose is taken up into the intracellular compartment. Consequently, a change of glucose concentration in 3 different compartments can contribute to the signal changes: (1) the intravascular space, (2) the EES, and (3) the intracellular space.

As a result, glucose-enhanced MR imaging is in principle able to visualize both perfusion effects (glucose flooding via the vessels) and intracellular metabolic processes. Though, latest results in DGE MR imaging brain tumor studies indicate a major contribution of BBB leakage and tissue perfusion.[16,18,30] Furthermore, both CEST and CESL may be additionally altered by pH, since an acidic tumor microenvironment can enhance DGE signals through proton exchange rate modulation.[31] Further studies in larger study samples are necessary in order to further evaluate the origin of the measured glucose signal and the potential benefit for clinical routine.

Fig. 1. Chemical proton exchange as the basis for glucose-enhanced MR imaging. Chemical proton exchange: the spontaneous exchange of metabolite-bound protons (here 5 hydroxyl groups of D-glucose) and the protons of free bulk water is the common physical principle of glucose-enhanced MR imaging approaches. The indirect detection via the water proton signal yields strong signal amplification proportional to the local glucose concentration.

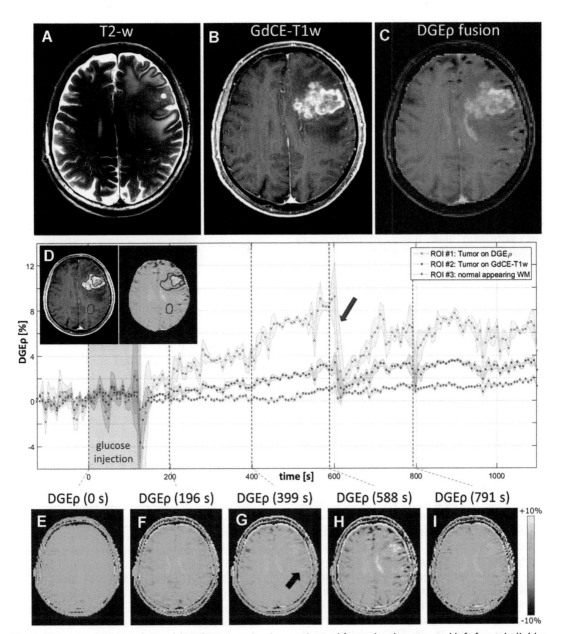

Fig. 2. Dynamic glucose-enhanced (DGE) MR imaging in a patient with previously untreated left-frontal glioblas-toma using the CESL-based DGE MR imaging technique. (*A*) T2-weighted (T2-w), (*B*) gadolinium-enhanced T1-w (GdCE-T1w), and (*C*) glucose-enhanced MR imaging based on T1ρ-weighted CESL imaging (DGEρ). Increased glucose-enhanced signal can be observed in the tumor region and in the (para-) ventricular area. Note an addi-tional hyperintense region located dorsal of the tumor area (*black arrow*) (*G*), not discernible in the GdCE-T1w image (*B*). (*D*) DGEρ time curves with a temporal resolution of 7 sec shown in the tumor region (ROI #1) and normal-appearing white matter (ROI #2). Continuously increasing DGEρ values can be observed in the tumor ROI following glucose injection. The red arrow marks an abrupt signal drop induced by patient motion. (*E–I*) DGEρ images (average of 5 consecutive images) at different time points after glucose injection. ROI, region of interest. (*From* Schuenke P, Paech D, Koehler C, et al. Fast and Quantitative T1ρ-Weighted Dynamic Glucose Enhanced MRI. Scientific Reports 2017;7(42093).)

TRANSLATION OF DYNAMIC GLUCOSE-ENHANCED MR IMAGING TO CLINICAL FIELD STRENGTH AT 3T

Recently, the feasibility of glucose-enhanced CE-sensitive MR imaging has also been demonstrated at clinical field strength of 3T by Herz and colleagues using CESL MR imaging[32] and by Xu and colleagues using the CEST approach.[33] Because of the small effect sizes, it is currently in question if a robust approach can be established at field strengths less than 7T. Consequently, DGE MR imaging may gain further attention for clinical applications in the near future, as the number of ultrahigh field MR imaging sites is continuously increasing and many with regulatory approval for limited clinical imaging.

NONMETABOLIZABLE GLUCOSE ANALOGUES FOR TUMOR IMAGING

Tumors have increased energy demand due to high cell proliferation and inefficient energy metabolism.[34–36] This characteristic has been used for diagnosis, staging, and therapy monitoring of multiple cancer types through PET using 18F-fluoro-deoxyglucose (^{18}F-FDG) for several decades.[37,38] Nonradioactive glucose analogues, for instance 2-deoxy-D-glucose (2DG) and 3-O-Methyl-D-glucose (3-OMG), undergo facilitated transit through glucose transporters in the cell membrane, similar to ^{18}F-FDG agents.[39] In animal tumor models it could be shown that 2DG[25] and 3-OMG[40,41] can act as a CEST and CESL contrast agent for brain tumor detection. Unlike natural D-Glucose, these analogues are nonmetabolizable, resulting in intracellular accumulation. Consequently, CEST or CESL imaging with 2DG or 3-OMG should yield larger signal contributions from the intracellular department compared with natural D-glucose and are therefore expected to have stronger weighting of glucose transport and metabolism, similar to ^{18}F-FDG agents.[25,30] 3-OMG may be a possible candidate for human application, whereas 2DG cannot be translated into clinical use due to its known toxicity.

REFERENCES

1. Radbruch A, Weberling LD, Kieslich PJ, et al. Gadolinium retention in the dentate nucleus and globus pallidus is dependent on the class of contrast agent. Radiology 2015;275:783–91.
2. Kanda T, Ishii K, Kawaguchi H, et al. High Signal Intensity in the Dentate Nucleus and Globus Pallidus on Unenhanced T1-weighted MR Images: Relationship with Increasing Cumulative Dose of a Gadolinium-based Contrast. Mater Radiol 2014; 270:834–41.
3. Kanda T, Osawa M, Oba H, et al. High signal intensity in dentate nucleus on unenhanced T1-weighted MR images: association with linear versus macrocyclic gadolinium chelate administration. Radiology 2015;275:803–9.
4. McDonald RJ, McDonald JS, Kallmes DF, et al. Intracranial Gadolinium Deposition after Contrast-enhanced MR Imaging. Radiology 2015;275: 772–82.
5. Radbruch A, Haase R, Kickingereder P, et al. Pediatric brain: no increased signal intensity in the dentate nucleus on unenhanced T1-weighted MR Images after consecutive exposure to a macrocyclic gadolinium-based contrast agent. Radiology 2017; 283:828–36.
6. Radbruch A. Are some agents less likely to deposit gadolinium in the brain? Magn Reson Imaging 2016; 34:1351–4.
7. Thomsen HS, Morcos SK, Almén T, et al. Nephrogenic systemic fibrosis and gadolinium-based contrast media: updated ESUR Contrast Medium Safety Committee guidelines. Eur Radiol 2012;23: 307–18.
8. Schuenke P, Koehler C, Korzowski A, et al. Adiabatically prepared spin-lock approach for T1ρ-based dynamic glucose enhanced MRI at ultrahigh fields. Magn Reson Med 2017;78:215–25.
9. Jones CK, Huang A, Xu J, et al. Nuclear Overhauser enhancement (NOE) imaging in the human brain at 7T. Neuroimage 2013;77:114–24.
10. Jin T, Wang P, Zong X, et al. MR imaging of the amide-proton transfer effect and the pH-insensitive nuclear overhauser effect at 9.4 T. Magn Reson Med 2013;69:760–70.
11. Zhou J, Payen J-F, Wilson DA, et al. Using the amide proton signals of intracellular proteins and peptides to detect pH effects in MRI. Nat Med 2003;9: 1085–90.
12. Haris M, Nanga RPR, Singh A, et al. Exchange rates of creatine kinase metabolites: feasibility of imaging creatine by chemical exchange saturation transfer MRI. NMR Biomed 2012;25:1305–9.
13. Haris M, Singh A, Cai K, et al. A technique for in vivo mapping of myocardial creatine kinase metabolism. Nat Med 2014;20:209.
14. Cai K, Haris M, Singh A, et al. Magnetic resonance imaging of glutamate. Nat Med 2012;18:302–6.
15. Roalf DR, Nanga RPR, Rupert PE, et al. Glutamate imaging (GluCEST) reveals lower brain GluCEST contrast in patients on the psychosis spectrum. Mol Psychiatry 2017;22:1298.
16. Paech D, Schuenke P, Koehler C, et al. T1ρ-weighted dynamic glucose-enhanced mr imaging in the human brain. Radiology 2017;285: 914–22.

17. Walker-Samuel S, Ramasawmy R, Torrealdea F, et al. In vivo imaging of glucose uptake and metabolism in tumors. Nat Med 2013;19:1067–72.

18. Xu X, Yadav NN, Knutsson L, et al. Dynamic Glucose-Enhanced (DGE) MRI: Translation to Human Scanning and First Results in Glioma Patients. Tomography 2015;1:105.

19. Chan KWY, McMahon MT, Kato Y, et al. Natural D-glucose as a biodegradable MRI contrast agent for detecting cancer. Magn Reson Med 2012;68: 1764–73.

20. Rivlin M, Horev J, Tsarfaty I, et al. Molecular imaging of tumors and metastases using chemical exchange saturation transfer (CEST) MRI. Sci Rep 2013;3: 3045.

21. Nasrallah FA, Pages G, Kuchel PW, et al. Imaging brain deoxyglucose uptake and metabolism by glucoCEST MRI. J Cereb Blood Flow Metab 2013;33: 1270–8.

22. Xu X, Chan KWY, Knutsson L, et al. Dynamic glucose enhanced (DGE) MRI for combined imaging of blood-brain barrier break down and increased blood volume in brain cancer. Magn Reson Med 2015;74:1556–63.

23. Jin T, Mehrens H, Hendrich KS, et al. Mapping Brain Glucose Uptake with Chemical Exchange-Sensitive Spin-Lock Magnetic Resonance Imaging. J Cereb Blood Flow Metab 2014;34:1402–10.

24. Zu Z, Spear J, Li H, et al. Measurement of regional cerebral glucose uptake by magnetic resonance spin-lock imaging. Magn Reson Imaging 2014;32: 1078–84.

25. Jin T, Mehrens H, Wang P, et al. Glucose metabolism-weighted imaging with chemical exchange-sensitive MRI of 2-deoxyglucose (2DG) in brain: Sensitivity and biological sources. NeuroImage 2016;143:82–90.

26. Zaiss M, Herz K, Deshmane A, et al. Possible artifacts in dynamic CEST MRI due to motion and field alterations. J Magn Reson 2019;298:16–22.

27. Boyd PS, Breitling J, Zimmermann F, et al. Dynamic glucose-enhanced (DGE) MRI in the human brain at 7 T with reduced motion-induced artifacts based on quantitative R1ρ mapping. Magn Reson Med 2020; 84:182–91.

28. Schuenke P, Paech D, Koehler C, et al. Fast and quantitative T1ρ-weighted dynamic glucose enhanced MRI. Sci Rep 2017;7:42093.

29. Knutsson L, Seidemo A, Rydhög Scherman A, et al. Arterial input functions and tissue response curves in dynamic glucose-enhanced (DGE) imaging: comparison between glucoCEST and blood glucose sampling in humans. Tomography 2018;4:164–71.

30. Tao J, Bistra I, Kevin HT, et al. Chemical exchange–sensitive spin-lock (CESL) MRI of glucose and analogs in brain tumors. Magn Reson Med 2018;80: 488–95.

31. Paech D, Radbruch A. CEST, pH, and Glucose Imaging as Markers for Hypoxia and Malignant Transformation. In: Pope W, editor. Glioma Imaging. Springer, Cham; 2020. https://doi.org/10.1007/978-3-030-27359-0_10.

32. Herz K, Lindig T, Deshmane A, et al. T1ρ-based dynamic glucose-enhanced (DGEρ) MRI at 3 T: method development and early clinical experience in the human brain. Magn Reson Med 2019;82: 1832–47.

33. Xu X, Sehgal AA, Yadav NN, et al. d-glucose weighted chemical exchange saturation transfer (glucoCEST)-based dynamic glucose enhanced (DGE) MRI at 3T: early experience in healthy volunteers and brain tumor patients. Magn Reson Med 2020;84:247–62.

34. Warburg O. On the origin of cancer cells. Science 1956;123:309–14.

35. Warburg O, Wind F, Negelein E. The metabolism of tumors in the body. J Gen Physiol 1927;8:519.

36. Agnihotri S, Zadeh G. Metabolic reprogramming in glioblastoma: the influence of cancer metabolism on epigenetics and unanswered questions. Neuro Oncol 2015;18:160–72.

37. Gambhir SS. Molecular imaging of cancer with positron emission tomography. Nat Rev Cancer 2002;2: 683–93.

38. Weber WA, Schwaiger M, Avril N. Quantitative assessment of tumor metabolism using FDG-PET imaging. Nucl Med Biol 2000;27:683 7.

39. Nakanishi H, Cruz NF, Adachi K, et al. Influence of glucose supply and demand on determination of brain glucose content with labeled methylglucose. J Cereb Blood Flow Metab 1996;16:439–49.

40. Sehgal AA, Li Y, Lal B, et al. CEST MRI of 3-O-methyl-D-glucose uptake and accumulation in brain tumors. Magn Reson Med 2019;81(3):1993–2000.

41. Zu Z, Jiang X, Xu J, et al. Spin-lock imaging of 3-o-methyl-D glucose (3oMG) in brain tumors. Magn Reson Med 2018;80:1110–7.

7-T Magnetic Resonance Imaging in the Management of Brain Tumors

Melanie A. Morrison, PhD, Janine M. Lupo, PhD*

KEYWORDS

- Ultrahigh-field MR imaging • Brain tumors • Glioma • Magnetic resonance spectroscopy • CEST
- Susceptibility-weighted imaging • Late effects

KEY POINTS

- Ultrahigh-field 7T magnetic resonance (MR) imaging is advantageous in providing new information that is complementary to the current capabilities of clinical systems.
- The progress of 7T MRI remains limited by patient contraindications and technical challenges caused by nonuniform fields, tissue heating and magnetic susceptibility artifacts.
- As more 7T scanners become available, additional studies are likely to emerge that will determine advantages of ultrahigh-field imaging for brain tumor management in the clinic.

INTRODUCTION

Brain cancer remains one of most fatal diseases affecting children and adults worldwide.[1] Characterized by the presence of 1 or more brain neoplasms, patients diagnosed with the disease experience poor prognoses and high mortalities caused by the rapid growth, heterogeneity, and unpredictable behavior that is often observed in many of these lesions. Although substantial progress has been made in terms of their management through technological advancements and research discoveries, therapeutic strategies have been relatively constant over the last decade, involving some combination of surgery, chemotherapy, and/or radiation therapy; the recent addition of wearable tumor-treating fields[2]; and, for certain nonmalignant tumors with slow growth characteristics, a surveillance approach.

Imaging, specifically magnetic resonance (MR) imaging at lower field strengths (1.5 T and 3 T), plays an integral role in the current management of brain tumors from diagnosis to treatment and posttherapeutic surveillance. However, growing evidence of the limited diagnostic accuracy of conventional imaging for brain tumors, namely contrast-enhanced (CE) T1-weighted (T1w), T2-weighted (T2w) fast spin-echo (FSE) and T2w FLAIR (fluid-attenuated inversion-recovery) imaging, has led to the exploitation of advanced MR imaging techniques (ie, spectroscopic, diffusion, perfusion, susceptibility-weighted, and functional imaging) to develop and validate robust imaging biomarkers for improved tissue characterization, and assessment of tumor progression and malignant transformation. The ability of imaging biomarkers to noninvasively capture physiologic and structural tumor features that reflect the underlying glioma biology is particularly advantageous because it could help better inform treatment strategies, including the appropriate timing for intervention.

Recent advancements in imaging technology leading to the emergence of state-of-the-art ultrahigh-field (UHF) MR imaging scanners ($\geq$7 T) has provided the opportunity to improve current management strategies for brain tumors through augmentation of both conventional and advanced MR imaging. Compared with lower field strengths, UHF MR imaging achieves higher signal-to-noise

Department of Radiology and Biomedical Imaging, University of California, San Francisco, 505 Parnassus Avenue, San Francisco, CA 94143, USA
* Corresponding author. Byers Hall UCSF, Box 2532, 1700 4th Street, Suite 303D, San Francisco, CA 94158-2330.
E-mail address: janine.lupo@ucsf.edu

Magn Reson Imaging Clin N Am 29 (2021) 83–102
https://doi.org/10.1016/j.mric.2020.09.007
1064-9689/21/© 2020 Elsevier Inc. All rights reserved.

ratio (SNR), enhanced susceptibility contrast, and improved contrast-to-noise ratio (CNR) that can be exploited to attain superior anatomic resolution, higher spatial and spectral specificity of advanced quantitative techniques, greater brain coverage, and shorter scan times.[3–5] When applied clinically, these benefits translate to increased detection sensitivity, including more accurate tumor delineation, higher inter-rater agreement, and ultimately improved diagnostic and surgical confidence to inform decision making.[5,6] Several prior studies in patients with brain tumors[4,7,8] and from other clinical populations[9–13] have repeatedly shown improvements in diagnostic accuracy when using UHF versus lower-field clinical images, echoing the enormous potential of UHF MR imaging in clinical applications.[6]

Since its inception in the late 1990s,[14] UHF imaging has seen expansive growth, having been pioneered for clinical use and developed to a mature enough stage where efficacy and feasibility are now warranted, but requiring more thorough validation in practice. Evidence of this growth comes from the more than 80 7-T scanners installed worldwide for human imaging over the last 2 decades,[3,15] along with the growing number of National Institutes of Health (NIH)–funded 7-T clinical investigations, and, more recently, US Food and Drug Administration (FDA) approval for the first 7-T scanner manufactured by Siemens Healthcare (Magnetom Terra; Erlangen, Germany).[16]

This article includes a discussion of the current status of 7-T MR imaging in the management of brain tumors across the pretherapeutic, peritherapeutic, and posttherapeutic stages, including its foreseeable role in tumor characterization and diagnosis; radiotherapy (RT) and neurosurgical planning; and assessment of treatment response, progression, and long-term treatment side effects.

PRETHERAPEUTIC
Novel Features on Conventional Imaging at Ultrahigh Field

To date, radiological diagnosis and initial histopathologic characterization of brain tumors to inform treatment strategy has largely relied on CE T1w, T2w, and FLAIR imaging. However, the diagnostic accuracy of these conventional imaging approaches is limited by their poor biological specificity of signal, and, furthermore, at clinical field strengths, by their lower SNR and achievable anatomic resolution. For example, clinical indictors of a higher-grade tumor with malignant features include the appearance of contrast enhancement on T1w images (caused by

disruption of the blood-brain barrier) and edema on FLAIR images (caused by swelling and accumulation of water in brain parenchyma). However, T2w FLAIR signal cannot distinguish between areas of edema and infiltrating tumor,[17] and some lower-grade tumors have the propensity to show contrast enhancement on T1w imaging, leading to erroneous diagnoses.[18,19] The inability to resolve finer anatomic structures because of resolution and SNR constraints can also limit sensitivity for intratumoral features and newly appearing metastatic brain lesions.

In UHF MR imaging, conventional imaging for brain tumors has been focused on the development of rapid anatomic images in order to avoid the need for multiple scans, while allowing patients and their treating teams to take advantage of the benefits of additional conventional and advanced MR imaging sequences with higher resolution and/or new quantitative, functional, and physiologic information.[7,8,20,21] Moenninghoff and colleagues[8] first compared T1w and T2w images acquired at 1.5 T and 7 T in 15 untreated but histologically proven astrocytomas (World Health Organization [WHO] grade II–IV), and found visually similar ring patterns of contrast enhancement after gadolinium (Gd) administration. They also reported that T2w 7-T images provided sharper delineation of central and peripheral intratumoral necrosis in a patient with glioblastoma (GBM; WHO grade IV).

Noebauer-Huhmann and colleagues[7] later compared contrast enhancement at 3 T versus 7 T after a half and full standard Gd dose using quantitative measures of tumor-to-brain contrast and lesion enhancement (difference in lesion signal before and after Gd administration). In 10 patients with either primary brain tumors or brain metastases they reported significantly higher tumor-to-brain contrast and lesion enhancement on 7-T T1w images at both half and full dose. Half-dose images at 7 T were superior to full-dose images at 3 T, suggesting the possibility of a dose reduction with clinical use of UHF scanners. More recently, Jakary and colleagues[21] compared clinical 3-T sequences and 7-T sequences optimized to match 3-T contrast, resolution, and scan time, and confirmed that half-dose Gd CE T1w and T2w 7-T images produce better lesion contrast and enhancement based on qualitative assessment by a senior neuroradiologist. However, when matched to clinical imaging parameters at 3 T, 7-T FLAIR images were found to be less robust for clinical use. An example of a clinical imaging protocol obtained at 7 T compared with 3 T is shown in **Fig. 1**. Around the same time, Springer and colleagues[6] used 10-point scale diagnostic confidence scores (DCSs) to

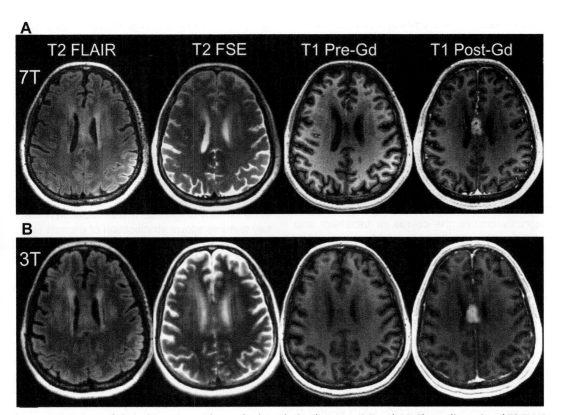

Fig. 1. Comparison of clinical imaging with matched resolution between 3 T and 7 T. Three-dimensional T2 FLAIR, FSE, and T1 inversion recovery spoiled gradient recalled precontrast and postcontrast images at 7 T (*A*) and 3 T (*B*) for a grade II glioma that progressed.

compare neuroradiologist evaluation of tumor characteristics (intracranial location, degree of malignancy, multiplicity) on 3-T versus 7-T conventional imaging, and reported slightly higher DCS for evaluation based on 7-T versus 3-T images, along with higher inter-rater agreement (87.9% at 7 T vs 75.8% at 3 T). Although their study did not use contrast agents or report DCSs for specific sequences, it did report higher SNR and CNR of 7-T images after correcting for differences in voxel size across field strengths. The study also highlighted the utility of 7-T T2*w gradient echo (GRE) images, along with using the phase signal to create susceptibility-weighted imaging (SWI) for enhanced visualization of neoangiogenesis in malignant tumors and corroborated similar 8-T human and postmortem studies of T2w FSE, T2*w GRE, and SWI images in gliomas.[22,23]

Although clinically equivalent 7-T FLAIR images have been found to provide no added diagnostic value,[21] when leveraging the SNR and resolution benefits of UHF imaging and using advance pulse sequence techniques such as magnetization preparation and hyperechoes, very-high-resolution

FLAIR images can be acquired to reveal new cortical features within clinically acceptable scan times (axial FLAIR images with in-plane resolutions of 0.57 × 0.57 mm^2 have been reported,[24] along with volumetric sequences that can achieve isotropic or near-isotropic resolutions ranging 0.5–0.8 mm^3 [6,25,26]). Notably, the enhanced appearance of a hyperintense rim corresponding with cortical layers I through III at the pial surface and ependyma around the ventricles has been reported by several studies as having the potential to aid radiological interpretation of intracortical lesions or lesions at the ventricular boundary.[6,26,27]

In a postmortem imaging study at 7 T, Van Veluw and colleagues[26] removed part of cortical layer I and found that the hyperintense rim disappeared in the area where it was removed on repeat imaging. The investigators noted that, in addition to the smaller voxel size of 7-T FLAIR images, as well as water diffusion from the cerebrospinal fluid (CSF), a longer T2 relaxation time constant at UHF is the likely contributor to this enhanced FLAIR feature. Further evidence of the contribution of CSF comes from a case study of a 21-year-old patient with a tectal glioma causing severe hydrocephalus, whereby preoperative FLAIR imaging at 7 T showed a thick hyperintense rim in the anterior lateral ventricles that depreciated on imaging following an endoscopic third ventriculostomy procedure to restore CSF flow.[27]

Histopathologic and Molecular Characterization of Gliomas for Stratification

With gliomas representing the most common primary brain tumor in adults, there has been a concerted effort over the years to overcome significant challenges associated with their management. In the pretherapeutic stage where initial diagnosis occurs, the course of treatment and outcome relies heavily on the ability to accurately characterize these tumors according to their histopathologic and molecular features. Although surgical biopsy can provide a confirmatory diagnosis, there is reluctance to submit patients to invasive procedures, especially those with slower-growing lesions that do not require upfront therapy. Biopsies are also limited in their ability to capture tumor spatial heterogeneity and could therefore lead to underestimation of disease severity.

Historically, gliomas have been grouped according to their histopathologic characteristics as either lower-grade glioma (LGG; WHO grades I–II) or high-grade glioma (HGG; WHO III–IV). However, in recent years this stratification approach has evolved with advances in molecular and genetic classification, highlighting the prognostic role of molecular signatures in the prediction of glioma behavior. This major paradigm shift in the management of glioma, marked by recent revision of the WHO diagnostic criteria to incorporate molecular features,[28] has been accompanied by a growing number of investigations leveraging quantitative and physiologic MR imaging methods to develop surrogate imaging biomarkers.

Two primary molecular features have been identified under the new WHO classification criteria: (1) somatic mutation status of isocitrate dehydrogenase (IDH) enzymes involved in energy production and biosynthesis, and (2) codeletion status of short-arm chromosome 1 and long-arm chromosome 19 (1p/19q) in tumor suppressor genes.[28] Mutation status of transcriptional regulator ATRX (alpha-thalassemia/mental retardation, X-linked) and TP53, a tumor suppressor gene, were found to be similarly diagnostic. Joint evaluation of these key features allows stratification of gliomas into 5 molecular subtypes, each of which is associated with a different median survival time despite some shared histopathologic characteristics (Table 1). Broadly, IDH wild-type (Wt) gliomas, which include WHO grades II and III pre-GBM astrocytomas and primary GBMs, are the most aggressive tumor types associated with the worst prognoses. IDH-mutated gliomas include WHO grades II and III oligodendrogliomas and presecondary GBM astrocytomas, the former having slightly better prognoses, and the latter ultimately transforming into secondary GBMs, but have an overall median survival longer than that of their IDH-Wt counterparts. Oligodendrogliomas are unique in that they are highly vascularized lesions similar to the more aggressive IDH-Wt gliomas, and therefore can easily confound noninvasive stratification based on imaging markers of blood flow, blood volume, or vascular density.[29]

At clinical field strengths, promising quantitative imaging biomarkers of glioma molecular status

Table 1
World Health Organization 2016 molecular subtypes of gliomas with differing prognoses

WHO Grade	Tumor Type	IDH Mutated	1p/19q Codeletion	ARTX Mutated	TP53 Mutated	Behavior/Prognosis
II/III	Oligodendroglioma	Yes	Yes	No	No	12–14-y median survival (grade II/III); >14 y (grade II)
II/III	Astrocytoma	Yes	No	Yes	Yes	Transforms to secondary GBM 3–8-y median survival
II/III	Astrocytoma	No	No	No	Yes	Pre-GBM; <16-mo median survival[30]
IV	GBM	Yes	No	Often	Often	Secondary GBM <31-mo median survival[31]
IV	GBM	No	No	No	No	Primary GBM <15-mo median survival[31]

Data from Refs.[30,31]

and/or tumor grade have been identified using advanced diffusion,[32–35] perfusion,[36–38] and spectroscopic[39–44] imaging techniques. Qualitative imaging biomarkers have furthermore been derived from susceptibility-weighted imaging (SWI)[45] and conventional T1w, T2w, and FLAIR imaging.[46–48] However, at UHF strengths, imaging biomarker development for glioma stratification has been centered on MR spectroscopic imaging (MRSI), chemical exchange saturation transfer (CEST) imaging, and SWI, given the added benefits of heightened SNR, improved spectral resolution, and enhanced susceptibility contrast,[3,5] as described later.

Magnetic resonance spectroscopic imaging

In vivo MRSI is a technique through which the presence and concentration of intratumoral and extratumoral metabolites can be quantified based on the frequency spectrum of the free induction decay or spin-echo–recovered ^1H or non-^1H (eg, phosphorus [^{31}P], carbon [^{13}C]) signal. Tumor metabolic processes and signatures are inferred by comparing spectra derived from within the tumor with that of the surrounding normal brain tissue. Specific characterization of gliomas using MRS at lower field strengths dates back to the emergence of localized spectroscopic acquisitions in the early 1990s. Since then, especially over the last decade with the overcoming of technical challenges (acquisition time, power deposition, field inhomogeneity),[49–51] gliomas have been associated with numerous signal alterations in metabolites such as N-acetyl aspartate (NAA), choline-containing compounds (Cho), creatine (Cr), lactate, lipid, myo-inositol (ml), glutamate (Glu), and 2-hydroxyglutarate (2HG). Neurobiologically, these metabolite-specific signal alterations are associated with an array of tumor metabolic processes that reflect cell viability, density, proliferation, energy expenditure, anaerobic glycolysis, and necrosis.[52,53]

With improved water suppression pulses and high-order shimming techniques designed for UHF, performing MRSI at increasing field strengths substantially increases the number of short-echo metabolites and accuracy of detectable long-echo metabolites (Fig. 2).[54,55] The latter is because, at 7 T, the T2 relaxation times of water, NAA, and creatine are shorter than those at 3 T, which allows them to fully relax between excitations, whereas T1 relaxation times increase with increase in field strength.[56–58] Lower-concentration, overlapping shorter-echo-time metabolites such as Glu, ml, taurine, scylloinositol, and glucose are also better visualized and discriminated at 7 T compared with lower field

strengths.[5,59–61] Such improvements in the accuracy and reliability of metabolite signal alterations measured at UHF further advance the technique toward a potential role in noninvasive molecular and histopathologic tumor characterization.

Detection of the 2HG metabolite, the first genetic mutation–specific imaging marker of the IDH mutation,[39–43] has been the central focus of most UHF MSRI studies of gliomas to date. Under healthy brain conditions, the intramitochondrial and extramitochondrial IDH enzymes catalyze the conversion of isocitrate to α-ketoglutarate. When gliomas carry the IDH mutation, cellular α-ketoglutarate undergoes further catalytic reduction to 2HG.[43] Because the 2HG metabolite is not found in normal or IDH-Wt tumor cells, it serves as a unique oncomarker of glioma molecular status.

Lazovic and colleagues[62] performed one of the early preclinical in vivo MRSI studies in 2012, validating 2HG and its link to the IDH mutation. Using a 7-T Bruker system, they imaged mice injected with human U87 glioma cells overexpressing either the mutated or Wt IDH enzymes, and reported in the former a 2HG resonance peak at 2.25 ppm (parts per million) coupled with significant reductions in Glu resonance between 2.31 and 2.35 ppm. This reduction in Glu was thought to represent the compromised oxidative metabolism, increased use of Glu in the citric acid cycle, and/or its irreversible conversion into 2HG. Quantification of 2HG at 7 T had proved to be valuable in distinguishing neighboring 2HG and Glu resonance peaks, a previous limitation of 2HG detection with MRSI at lower clinical field strengths.

Around the same time, results from the first 7-T human studies of 2HG were surfacing,[40,63–67] with multiple groups trending toward the use of long echo times (75–110 milliseconds) to improve discrimination of the 2HG resonance peak from Glu and other neighboring metabolites. Longer echo times effectively attenuate complex signals from macromolecules and narrow the spectral line width of neighboring peaks in a multiplet, thereby enhancing their separation.

Poptani and colleagues[68] were the first to use a two-dimensional (2D) MSRI approach to detect 2HG in IDH mutant gliomas. Specifically, they used a 2D localized correlated spectroscopy sequence that exploits cross-peak resonances to detect 2HG without limiting quantification of other useful metabolites for glioma characterization. At UHF strengths, the spectral resolution of cross-peaks improves substantially with the accompanied increase in SNR. More recently, Choi and colleagues[69] showcased a novel

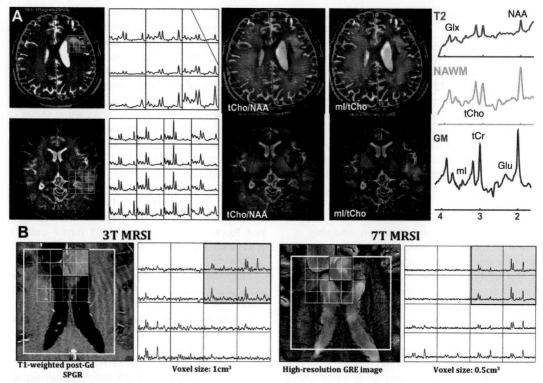

Fig. 2. (*A*) Short-echo, spin-echo MRSI at 7 T, corresponding maps of total Cho (tCho)/NAA and mI/tCho, and example spectra from a gray matter, white matter, and T2 lesion voxel for 2 patients with treated gliomas. (*B*) Increased SNR and spectral resolution available at 7 T allow higher resolution of metabolite maps and improved quantification of long-echo metabolites.

DRAG-EPSI (dual-read out alternated gradients echo-planar spectroscopic imaging) approach for time-efficient and reliable high-resolution 2HG imaging at 7 T, whereas Scheffler and colleagues[70] reported the first demonstration of MRSI of 2HG at 9.4 T. The ratio of 2HG/Cho (and mI/Cho) when quantified at 7 T can aid more precise IDH classification of gliomas into either predominate IDH1 (extramitochondrial) or IDH2 (intramitochondrial) mutated gliomas.[71] However, despite the clear prognostic value of 2HG and the advantage of UHF MR imaging for its in vivo quantification, validation studies are needed with larger sample sizes (>20), along with a consensus on the optimal MRSI sequence for quantification of both 2HG and other cancer-related metabolites, before the technique will be suitable for widespread clinical use. As 7 T scanners become more frequently used for brain tumor imaging in the coming years, there will be more opportunities for validating these methods.

Fewer explorative UHF studies of gliomas have involved ^{1}H-MRSI of non-2HG metabolite ratios and ^{31}P-MRSI, a more challenging technique that generally yields lower sensitivity than ^{1}H-MRSI.[72]

Li and colleagues[58] imaged 29 patients with glioma (12 grade II, 10 grade III, 7 grade IV) using a less-conventional short-echo sequence and found significantly increased Cho-to-Cr ($P = .0137$) and decreased Glu-to-Cr ($P = .0012$) ratios in the grade II tumors. The investigators reported in a later study, comparing glioma metabolite profiles derived from short-echo versus long-echo sequences, that the former was most useful for serial evaluation of large, heterogeneous lesions given the benefit of increased sensitivity for multimetabolite detection.[73] Hangel and colleagues[74] recently reported on a patch-based, super-resolution reconstruction technique for improved multimetabolite mapping using MRSI at 7 T, resolving unpresented detail of complex metabolic density in heterogeneous gliomas that topographically agreed with tracer uptake on PET. Although the first UHF ^{31}P-MRSI results in a patient with glioma were acquired at 9.4 T,[75] Korzowski and colleagues[50,76] showed improvements in the mapping of pH values (ie, level of acidity in tissue) even at 7 T, where they were able to differentiate between intracellular and extracellular pH, and tumor versus normal-appearing brain tissue.

Chemical exchange saturation transfer imaging

Overcoming some of the limitations of MRSI, including reduced sensitivity caused by low metabolite concentrations and the need for longer scan times to achieve sufficient SNR, CEST MR imaging is a novel contrast technique that is capable of detecting low concentrations metabolites with significantly higher sensitivity than MRSI. This detection was achieved using standard MR imaging to continuously saturate and exchange protons between a chemical species of interest (with a ^1H proton in its structure) and surrounding water, resulting in a net decrease in water signal and an indirect measure of the species' concentration.

The technique was first introduced 2 decades ago by Ward and colleagues,[77] and a few years later it was discovered that the ^1H groups of amides in mobile proteins and peptides could be detected, providing a novel endogenous contrast reflecting tissue pH levels.[78] Coined amide proton transfer (APT) imaging, Zhou and colleagues,[79] who first reported on APT, imaged the first patient with glioma in the same year. APT imaging has since been performed at clinical field strengths for glioma detection and classification,[80–82] and more recently using UHF MR imaging.[83–86] These last studies found APT useful for differentiating glioma from normal-appearing tissue,[83] characterizing a glioma's proliferative potential and intratumoral bleeding,[85] and predicting overall and progression-free survival in newly diagnosed HGG.[84,86] Receiving equal attention in UHF studies is a similar technique called nuclear Overhauser enhancement (NOE) imaging,[87,88] which, through a more complex dipole transfer scheme,[88] can indirectly measure amide concentrations with greater sensitivity than APT. Heo and colleagues[83] performed APT and NOE imaging at 7 T in 10 patients with glioma (6 grade II, 2 grade III, and 2 grade IV) and found that, although both techniques reduced signal in the tumor regions relative to normal-appearing tissues, only the NOE signals were able to differentiate between low and high grades (II vs III and IV). More recently, amine CEST contrast (amines form amides through interactions with carboxylic acids) has also shown promise in discriminating 1p/19q codeletion status,[89,90] although this has yet to be explored in patients with brain tumors at 7 T.

Although CEST MR imaging holds promise in the preoperative characterization of tumor acidity and hypoxicity,[91] and shorter scan times compared with MRSI make it more attractive clinically, there still exist challenges that have limited its rapid adoption in the clinic, such as how to interpret the signal and its frequent contaminants.[92] With only a few UHF studies of gliomas primarily targeting amides but also other cancer biomarkers such as glutamate,[93] along with new evidence that CEST signal intensities at 7 T in HGG are anatomic location dependent,[94] more investigations are needed.

Susceptibility-weighted imaging

At UHF strengths, the magnetic susceptibility effect increases significantly, resulting in drastic improvements in T2*-weighted and phase contrast, as well as the ability to derive high-resolution SWI images with heightened contrast of vascular structures compared with lower field. SWI is a postprocessing technique that incorporates filtered phase information to enhance tissue contrast of T2*-weighted magnitude images, yielding superb visualization of cerebral veins and other iron-containing or blood-containing compounds, such as hemorrhage (**Fig. 3**). With abnormal changes in local brain vasculature representing a common feature of brain tumor aggressiveness, T2*-weighted imaging and SWI have been established as advantageous techniques for glioma characterization and the evaluation of posttreatment effects (discussed later).[95]

In 2 of the earlier proof-of-concept studies, Christoforidis and colleagues[22,23] acquired in vivo and postmortem T2*-weighted imaging on pathologically proven GBMs at 1.5 T and 8 T, along with digital subtraction angiography, demonstrating the exclusive ability of UHF images to resolve areas of abnormal microvascularity with high spatial resolution. Similarly, it was later shown by Moenninghoff and colleagues[8] in a larger cohort of 5 patients with pathologically proven astrocytomas (WHO grades II–IV) that T2w and T2*-weighted images acquired at 7 T outperformed those acquired at 1.5 T in terms of image contrast of presumed microvasculature and necrosis. Around the same time, only a few years after the first phase images were acquired in patients with brain tumors on clinical and UHF scanners,[96,97] a pivotal study by Li and colleagues[98] reported on the increased sensitivity of SWI compared with conventional T2w images (albeit at 3 T) for the detection of small vessels and microhemorrhages in astrocytomas. Since then, 2 notable studies have investigated the usefulness of UHF SWI images for glioma grading and IDH classification. The first was a study by Di leva and colleagues,[99] who, in 36 patients (5 grade II, 5 grade III, 22 grade IV), used computer-based, fractal image analysis to quantify intratumoral microbleeds and microvasculature from 7-T SWI in order to differentiate LGG from HGG (separated as a vs b and a vs d,

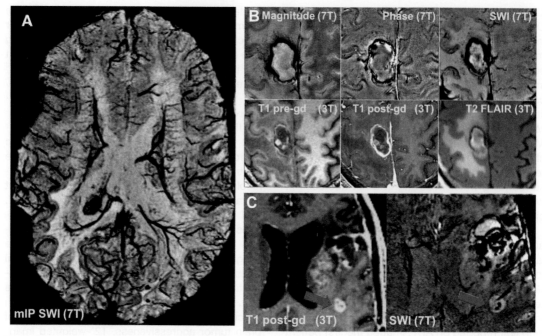

Fig. 3. Visualization of cerebral veins feeding an ependymoma (*A*) and other iron-containing or blood-containing compounds such as hemorrhage in a stable lesion (*B*) and recurrent tumor (*C, red arrows*) posttreatment.

where a = grades II, b = grades IV, d = grades II–III [unequivocal classification], III, and IV). They identified a trend of higher fractal dimension (the geometric complexity of intratumoral patterns) with increasing tumor grade, concluding that the 7 T was useful for detecting intratumoral vascular architectures.

The second study was performed by Grabner and colleagues[100] and involved measurement of the local image variance (LIV; a metric that increases with density of blood vessels) on 7-T SWI images in 30 patients diagnosed with a glioma. They contrasted LIV based on tumor grade (n_{LGG} = 9; LGG = grades II only), as well as IDH status ($n_{wildtype}$ = 15) and enhancement status ($n_{positive}$ = 13), and found significantly higher means (P<.0001) in the more aggressive glioma subtypes (ie, an HGG, IDH Wt, and/or CE lesion). Such findings, coupled with the ability to acquire 7-T SWI using rapid acquisition techniques that do not compromise vessel contrast,[101] hold potential for the future use of UHF SWI in the pretherapeutic stage, whether analyzed quantitatively or used for qualitative evaluation with conventional imaging.

Additional techniques

In addition to MRSI, CEST, and SWI, quantitative imaging of sodium (^{23}Na), as opposed to conventional proton (^{1}H) MR imaging, has recently been explored at UHF strengths in the context of classifying gliomas according their grade and IDH status, as well predicting tumor progression. The amount of sodium signal detected in a brain area reflects the underlying functional status of sodium channels and sodium-potassium pumps, which regulate cell proliferation, a key feature of tumorigenesis, thus making sodium imaging ideal for evaluating brain tumors. Biller and colleagues[102] found a significant correlation between the local sodium signal (normalized by total tissue Na), measured in 34 treatment-naive patients with a confirmed glioma (WHO grades I–IV), and tumor proliferation index (%Ki-67). Local signal was also capable of distinguishing IDH mutant from Wt tumors with an optimal cutoff that also predicted progression-free survival time with greater accuracy than IDH status alone. The investigators also used the sodium signal to discriminate between GBMs and other histologic glioma subtypes (ie, pilocytic astrocytoma, oligodendroglioma WHO grade II, anaplastic astrocytoma, anaplastic oligodendroglioma). A similar finding of ^{23}Na-facilitated discrimination of glioma tumor grade (LGG vs HGG) and genetic subtype (IDH and promotor methylation status) was reported by Paech and colleagues[103] in pilot study of 28 patients with glioma. Although sodium imaging of brain tumors and other indications is still in its infancy, lagging proton MR imaging and not yet having solidified a role in the clinic, the emergence of UHF studies showing significant improvements in SNR and acquisition time are leading the technique in the right direction.[104]

In addition, inflow-based vascular space occupancy (iVASO) perfusion MR imaging at 7 T,[105] a technique that provides quantitative measures of cerebral vascular hemodynamics based on the kinetics of exogenous and endogenous contrast agents in transit through the brain tissue,[106] has been compared with dynamic susceptibility contrast (DSC) perfusion imaging at 3 T in 12 patients with glioma. Intratumoral arteriolar cerebral blood volume (CBV_a) from 7-T iVASO was found to correlate with tumor grade ($r = 0.37$, $P = .04$) and trend with total-CBV derived from 3-T DSC imaging ($R^2 = 0.28$, $P = .07$) with comparable SNR. Although these findings reiterate the biomarker potential of CBV that has been shown in prior studies at clinical field strengths,[107–109] CBV measurements have not been widely exploited in UHF brain tumor studies, likely because of the additional susceptibility artifacts present in echo planar imaging (EPI) for DSC perfusion and longer T1s for dynamic CE perfusion.

Detection of Brain Metastases, Intracranial and Benign Skull-based Tumors

UHF MR imaging techniques have also proved to be advantageous in the management of various non–glial cell tumors, where there are unique challenges associated with early and accurate detection.[110] One such challenge lies in the detection of small brain metastases, which represent the most common malignancy affecting the brain.[3] Two groups have investigated the sensitivity of 7-T T1w images for small brain metastases: the first was a preclinical study of mice injected with cells derived from human melanoma brain metastases that reported the detection of lesions as small as 100 μm,[111] whereas the second found no difference in the detection rate of bronchial carcinoma brain metastases among 12 patients imaged at 1.5 and 7 T.[112] However, the investigators of the latter study did identify 20% more intralesional microhemorrhages when reviewing 7-T versus 1.5-T SWI images acquired in the same protocol. Because microscopic bleeding is a common feature of brain metastases, SWI holds promise for monitoring early vascular changes during the genesis of new metastatic lesions.[113]

MR imaging at 7 T has also been used to aid the detection of benign pituitary tumors that secrete excess cortisol into the body, leading to the development of Cushing disease, a rare condition with a broad spectrum of internal and external symptoms such as type 2 diabetes and excessive bruising.[114] Because these tumors are often difficult to appreciate on conventional clinical imaging and the alternative diagnostic test is an invasive procedure involving sinus sampling of cortisol levels, 7-T MR imaging may be a better alternative.[115] Law and colleagues[115] showed this in a case study of a 27-year-old woman with Cushing disease, whereby conventional imaging at 1.5 and 3 T, as well as 1.5-T dynamic contrast imaging, were negative. Sinus sampling suggested a right-sided pituitary microadenoma, which was thereafter confirmed on postcontrast 7-T MR imaging with characteristic focal hypoenhancement.[115]

In a larger study of 16 patients with clinically and biochemically proven Cushing disease,[116] 2 neuroradiologists reviewed precontrast and postcontrast T1w and T2w images from 1.5-T and 7-T MR imaging examinations in a random order to determine the presence or absence of a surgery-confirmed pituitary lesion. Although no difference in interobserver agreement was found across field strengths, 7-T MR imaging resulted in a different diagnosis for 7 patients (44%), including the detection of a lesion not seen at 1.5 T (4 out of 7 cases, 3 of which were surgically confirmed) and the refinement of lesion locations (3 out of 7 cases). Thus, requesting a 7-T MR imaging examination in the rare case of suspected Cushing disease could meaningfully alter patient management, allowing patients to forgo invasive sinus sampling and, in confirmed cases, aiding surgical planning.

Other cases where 7-T MR imaging has been useful for lesion characterization include (1) 2 orbital choroidal melanomas, for which the degree of optic nerve involvement could not be accurately depicted using clinical MR imaging alone[10]; (2) a benign cyst that appeared as a temporal mass and was diagnosed by ruling out parenchymal involvement and confirming enhancement arising from the choroid plexus[10]; as well as (3) skull-based tumors arising from the hippocampal region that are often affected by susceptibility artifacts but can be visualized using high-spatial-resolution 7-T FSE sequences with minimal artifact.[6] In line with these examples, 7 T could also be potentially advantageous in determining the extent of tumor infiltration in areas of edema, and differentiating between necrotic primary brain tumors, necrotic metastases, and cerebral abscesses.[117]

PERITHERAPEUTIC
Presurgical Planning

Surgical resection plays an integral role in the treatment of gliomas and other brain tumors, typically preceding radiation therapy and adjuvant chemotherapy for maximal therapeutic efficacy. Although gross total resection has been linked to more favorable patient outcomes,[118] maximizing the extent of resection remains challenged by the need to spare eloquent brain areas such that vital functions can be preserved. To achieve this dual goal, functional brain mapping techniques have become routinely used in standard practice. These techniques include direct cortical electrical stimulation (DCES), which allows real-time intraoperative mapping of eloquent brain areas while the patient is awake and performing motor and/or neurocognitive tasks during surgery.[119] Although DCES is considered the gold standard, it is limited in its ability to inform the craniotomy location, size, and surgical trajectory. Accordingly, noninvasive preoperative mapping of brain activity and white matter neuroanatomy (derived from functional MR [fMR] imaging and diffusion tensor imaging [DTI], respectively) are usually performed in conjunction with DCES to aid surgical planning, guidance, and confidence.[119]

Although a more thorough discussion of fMR imaging and the advantages of acquiring these data at UHF strengths is included elsewhere in this issue, the technique relies on temporal changes in T2*-weighted contrast to reveal local areas of neurovascular coupling in response to a patient's performance on a task or spontaneous fluctuations in brain activity that occur during rest. Although good reproducibility and spatial accuracy of activation patterns corresponding with motor and language function have previously been shown for fMR imaging data acquired at 3 T,[120,121] the overall reliability of the blood oxygenation level–dependent (BOLD) signal measured by fMR imaging still remains a subject of debate. UHF MR imaging presents an opportunity to enhance fMR imaging reliability, primarily through spatial and temporal SNR gains that increase sensitivity to the BOLD effect,[122,123] but also through other benefits, such as the observed reduction in sensitivity for larger draining veins classified as false-positive signal.[124,125] For example, Gizewski and colleagues[126] evaluated whole-brain fMR imaging data acquired at 1.5 and 7 T in 9 volunteers during a finger tapping task and found a 2-fold to 5-fold higher BOLD signal change in the 7-T data depending on the motor region, as well as activity in the thalamus that was rarely seen at 1.5 T.

Beisteiner and colleagues[127] similarly showed an increase in percentage signal change in 7-T versus 3-T data, larger activation volumes, and higher CNR during preoperative localization of the primary motor area in 17 patients. Although BOLD sensitivity was improved at 7 T in these studies, the data still suffered from common artifacts seen in UHF imaging, including reduced signal homogeneity, signal dropout, geometric distortions, and larger motion artifacts. Corrections for geometric distortions are especially critical in the context of using UHF images for treatment planning, because distortions of up to 5 mm have been observed in raw EPI data that could affect localization and have consequences for surgical planning.[128] These drawbacks make it unclear whether 7-T fMR imaging would offer a net clinical benefit compared with what is already provided by clinical imaging.

DTI, a technique that probes the brownian motion of water within tissue to yield microstructural information dominated by signal from the interstitial compartment, is similarly affected by field-related artifacts at 7 T that have limited its use to reconstruction of white matter tracts for surgical planning. Wen and colleagues[129] are the only group to have developed and applied a 7-T diffusion sequence in 20 patients with glioma, showing the ability to acquire 7-T DTI data that were equivalent to typical 3-T DTI protocols in terms of spatial resolution (2 mm isotropic), image quality, and scan time (<6 minutes) with 90 total diffusion directions acquired with 2 different b-values. Nonetheless, the performance of such data in a clinical setting to aid in surgical planning has yet been explored.

Radiotherapy Planning

Several groups have recently leveraged increases in spatial resolution with UHF imaging in order to improve the precision of RT planning in patients with brain tumors. Regnery and colleagues[24] compared the quality and utility of 3-T versus 7-T FLAIR images for RT planning in 15 patients with GBM and found that 7-T images showed greater white matter SNR and gray-to-white matter contrast, and reduced margins of the gross total treatment volume (even when 3 T and 7 T were acquired on the same day). Although the latter finding might suggest better visualization of the treatment boundary with 7-T images, the investigators admit that the difference could be attributed to lower image quality in the temporal lobes affecting discrimination of the edema from white matter where 7-T images had significantly lower edema-to-white matter contrast than 3T images.

In a phantom study by Peerlings and colleagues,[130] the investigators compared the geometric accuracy of 3-T and clinically optimized 7-T images for RT planning and found that the 7-T images carried a wider distribution of global and local geometric distortion values measured across 436 points of interest (range: 0.3–2.2 mm vs 0.2–0.8 mm [global], 0.2 to 1.2 mm versus 0.1 to 0.7 mm [local] for 7 T and 3 T, respectively). Nonetheless, most 7-T sequences (apart from the MPRAGE [magnetization-prepared rapid acquisition with gradient echo] sequence) resulted in clinically acceptable geometric distortions of less than or equal to 1 mm when measured within spherical volume diameters of up to 101.7 mm centered on the magnetic isocenter,[130] whereas volumes (eg, lesions and organs at risk [OARs]) residing outside the central brain in areas such as the frontal lobe, experienced greater distortion effects. One solution to overcome this clinical barrier is to incorporate local distortion into the safety margins for spatial treatment uncertainties. These estimates could perhaps be referenced from atlases designed for reproducible delineation of OARs[131] based on robust 7-T MR imaging sequences. Without a robust and reliable method to correct for distortions, including demonstration of performance in a large cohort in relation to outcomes, it is unlikely that 7-T MR imaging will become the standard for planning treatment interventions.

POSTTHERAPEUTIC
Monitoring Tumor Response to Therapy

Although there have been a wealth of studies in the literature on using various types of anatomic, physiologic, functional, and metabolic MR imaging techniques to identify the best candidates for novel therapies, provide early markers of response or progression, spatially monitor changes caused by different therapeutic regimens, and predict which patients are more likely to progress earlier and when, only a handful of studies have been reported at 7 T. The first dates back to 2012 when Grabner and colleagues[132] investigated changes in brain tumor vascularization during antiangiogenic therapy in the form of bevacizumab. By performing serial SWI and T1w imaging at baseline, 2 weeks, and 4 weeks after initiation of therapy in 5 adult patients with HGG, they found that the lesions completely resolved in 3 of 5 patients, whereas 1 patient experienced a rapid increase of lesion size despite therapy. SWI at 7 T showed progressive increase of irregular hypointense structures, most likely corresponding with increasing amounts of pathologic microvasculature at the time of progression, despite a prior study showing that more SWI hypointensity within the contrast-enhancing lesion at baseline was associated with a longer survival.[133] In another patient with progressive neurologic decline, 7-T images showed multiple intratumoral microhemorrhages after bevacizumab. Correlation of postmortem neuroimaging with histopathology confirmed that these hypointense structures identified on 7-T SWI corresponded to tumor vasculature. Although the feasibility of high-resolution imaging of intratumoral arteries has also been shown with 7-T time-of-flight (TOF) MR angiography (MRA), its utility in assessing antiangiogenic efficacy has not yet been studied.[110]

With the increased sensitivity to the CEST effect and sodium concentration at 7 T comes the potential ability to detect more subtle changes to treatment and earlier response assessment. Recent studies have shown the potential of NOE-mediated CEST imaging at 7 T in patients with HGG treated with conventional RT, where discrimination of future responders from nonresponders was possible immediately on completion of RT before changes were observed on conventional MR imaging.[134] CEST-derived contrasts, particularly NOE-weighted imaging and downfield-NOE-suppressed APT, were also able to significantly predict early progression after RT and chemotherapy in patients with GBM.[84] In addition to its role in diagnosing glioma subtype and prognosis, there is some evidence that sodium MR imaging at 7 T may also hold promise in monitoring response to therapy in patients with brain tumors, with increases in tissue sodium concentration measured at 7 T observed following stereotactic radiosurgery that were not visible on proton MR imaging, as reported in a recent case study.[135]

Later in a patient's disease trajectory, changes that are caused by the treatment inducing gliosis can often mimic the appearance of recurrent tumor on anatomic imaging. In ex vivo high-resolution MRS of image-guided tissue samples, the ratio of mI to Cho has shown great promise as a marker for distinguishing tumor progression from proliferation of reactive astrocytes in response to treatment at the time of suspected tumor progression.[136] On lower-field-strength clinical scanners, mI peaks often overlap with the peak of glycine, which is an inhibitory neurotransmitter. Decreases in mIG (sum of mI and glycine) relative to Cr from in vivo MRS data at 1.5 T were initially observed in high-grade astrocytomas compared with low-grade lesions.[137] At 7 T, mI has been successfully separated from glycine because of the increased SNR and dispersion of peaks.[58] This property facilitates the sensitivity to and quantification of mI and other short-echo metabolites, as shown by Li and colleagues[58] using short-echo MRSI at 7 T, who showed that increased mI to Cho was present in a stable lesion, whereas total choline to NAA was increased in pathologically confirmed recurrent glioma. Although these preliminary results are promising for the use of 7 T for this application, more studies need to be performed to validate these findings before they are ready for use in clinical practice.

Detection and Characterization of the Late Effects of Radiotherapy-induced Vascular Injury

One of the most studied late effects of RT on otherwise healthy brain tissue has been the associated vascular injury in the form of hemosiderin-containing cerebral microbleeds (CMBs). Although the initial appearance of these microhemorrhages on T2*-weighted imaging at lower field strengths dates back to the early 2000s, the higher susceptibility contrast and SNR available at higher fields strengths now allows clinicians to visualize CMBs as small as submillimeter in diameter with increased sensitivity and detect the formation of these lesions earlier in time than previously was possible.[138] SWI at 7 T additionally provides heightened contrast of CMBs to the surrounding brain tissue,[4,139] improving the performance of automated detection and segmentation tools for more robust quantification by increasing sensitivity compared with human raters and reducing the number of false-positives that have to be censored manually.[140–143] These advances along with more than a 10-fold reduction in human effort when applying them at 7 T have facilitated the monitoring of their formation and size over time after RT.[144,145]

Although larger CMBs can be visualized at even 1.5-T field strength scanners if a long enough echo time is used, several studies have shown the benefit in detection at 7 T for both T2*-weighted magnitude GRE images and on SWI.[4,139,146] Besides a reported 30% and up to 3-fold increase in total CMB counts compared with 3-T[4] and 1.5-T[139,146] SWI respectively, both intrarater and inter-rater variability in CMB counts was also significantly reduced at 7 T compared with lower field strengths.[139] The addition of multiple echoes and the ability to increase the resolution at 7 T within a reasonable scan time has afforded an extra 25% increase in CMB detection sensitivity on multiecho 7-T SWI compared with single-echo 7-T SWI images of the same in-plane resolution but acquired with twice the voxel thickness.[147] The multiple echoes and improved resolution also increased the conspicuity of smaller, low-

contrast CMBs, which are often missed by automated and human raters.[147] However, if CMBs are in an area prone to susceptibility artifacts (such as the temporal lobe) or iron deposition (as in the basal ganglia), their detection is more likely to be obscured at 7 T,[4,141,148] favoring a shorter echo time to detect lesions in these more inferior brain regions.[149]

Quantification of the formation of CMBs that result as a late-effect of RT-induced vascular injury was first reported by Lupo and colleagues[138] using 7-T SWI. This retrospective study in long-term stable adult patients who were treated with prior external beam RT for a glioma 2 to 17 years before the time of imaging revealed an onset of CMB formation in irradiated patients approximately 2 years after receiving radiation or combined chemoradiation therapy. This phenomenon was not observed in patients treated with chemotherapy only. The prevalence of these microbleeds increased as a function of time elapsed since treatment with radiation, as shown in **Fig. 4**A, and lesions that appeared later often extended outside of the T2-hyperintensity lesion and into the contralateral hemisphere. The large variation in the number of these lesions observed, both across patients and with time, was most likely caused by differences in radiation dose to normal tissue, because it has since been shown that CMBs form more frequently and sooner in regions that experienced a higher dose of radiation.[150] However, if enough time elapses, CMBs also arise from vasculature exposed to less than 30 Gy of radiation.[150] Similar findings were subsequently reported in a smaller study of 10 patients with LGG who received RT 12 to 36 months prior, whereby CMBs were observed in 7 out of 10 patients in regions that received a greater than 45-Gy dose of radiation.[151] In a subset of these patients that were scanned serially, some CMBs were found to resolve contemporaneous with new ones forming. The ability to serially visualize these effects on normal tissue along with radiation dose received within the same patient in a larger cohort will be important in assessing the long-term impact of radiation. This issue is of particular importance in patients with lower-grade tumors and longer survival.

A larger study by Morrison and colleagues[144] has since investigated risk factors for radiation-induced CMB formation and has tracked individual CMB characteristics over time. All 91 patients that were scanned at 1 year or more post-RT had CMBs, whereas only 4 of the 22 nonirradiated control patients presented with fewer than 5 CMBs each. The total number and volume of CMBs increased by 18% and 11% per year, respectively, although individual CMBs decreased in volume

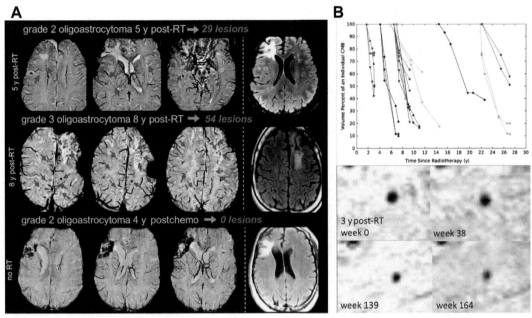

Fig. 4. (*A*) Increases in the number of RT-induced CMBs (*arrows*) with time since radiation. (*B*) Subsequent decreases in individual CMB size over time.

over time, as shown in **Fig. 4**B. Simultaneous to these microvascular changes, fractional anisotropy values of surrounding tissue decreased by a median of 6.5% per year. After accounting for age, time since RT, sex, and race, significant risk factors of CMB formation included a diagnosis of grade III anaplastic astrocytoma, frontal lobe tumor, and history of multiple surgical resections. Although this study shed light on potential clinical factors affecting the formation of radiation-induced CMBs, how their location and rate of formation relate to the known cognitive impairment experienced by this population has yet to be determined.

Two confounding factors present in these studies of adult gliomas are the variability in tumor location and the nonuniform radiation field to which normal brain tissue is exposed because of conforming focal radiation to these irregularly shaped lesions. These limitations make it difficult to examine regional sensitivity to radiation-induced injury and the effects on cognitive function when the tumor is in supratentorial brain tissue. However, children with medulloblastomas, provide a less variable model for studying radiation-induced vascular injury because they receive uniform whole-brain radiation of the same dose, typically survive well into adulthood, and have tumors within the posterior fossa or outside of the brain areas being analyzed. Using

7-T SWI, the authors were able to detect the onset of CMBs in 19 patients treated with whole-brain or focal RT 1 month to 20 years prior as early as 6 months following treatment, with 1 or more CMBs detected in all patients after 1 year post-RT.[152] Significantly more CMBs were present in patients who received whole-brain irradiation compared whole ventricular RT, with risk factors including RT type, a higher RT dose, increasing time since RT, and (unlike in adults) younger age during RT. Apart from RT dose, these factors were associated with impaired memory performance, and follow-up data in a subset of patients revealed increase in CMB formation with worsening verbal memory performance. Vascular injury was also found to affect the arteries in these patients, as quantified by three-dimensional TOF MRA, another sequence that greatly benefits from the increased SNR and contrast available at 7 T.[9] Patients treated with prior whole-brain RT as children had significantly lower arterial volumes and a higher proportion of smaller vessels compared with those who received whole-ventricular or no RT.[153] Arterial volume also decreased with CMB count and with worse verbal memory performance. Although these studies potentially provide a previously missing link between the extent of radiation-induced vascular injury and impact on cognitive function, they need to be validated in a larger cohort.

IMPRESSION AND SUMMARY

Although UHF MR imaging is advantageous in providing information that is complementary to the current capabilities of 1.5-T and 3-T systems, it remains to be seen whether it will replace state-of-the art 3-T scanners in the same way that 3 T has supplanted 1.5 T for brain tumor imaging. The progress of UHF imaging systems has been limited by technical challenges caused by nonuniform static (B0) and RF (B1) fields, higher specific absorption rates resulting in tissue heating, and magnetic susceptibility artifacts that still remain, despite numerous methodological advances to date. To optimally leverage the advantages and maximize the potential of UHF for clinical applications, diverse strategies need to be introduced, such as incorporating multitransmit developments that have been shown to mitigate field inhomogeneity into robust, user-friendly applications for routine clinical use. As more 7-T scanners become available and gain FDA 510(k) clearance, more confirmatory studies are likely to emerge in these areas, followed by larger, prospective, multicenter trials that will weigh the advantages of UHF imaging for brain tumor management against its disadvantages, including patient contraindications that cannot be overcome by technical strategies. The success of these systems will ultimately depend on the new information that can be attained that is not technologically possible at lower field systems, as opposed to incrementally improving the quality of the current 3-T standard.

CLINICS CARE POINTS

- 7T MRI significantly improves diagnostic sensitivity for brain tumors and post-treatment effects.
- Patients may experience more claustrophobia, dizziness, and/or peripheral nerve stimulation than during clinical MR imaging.

ACKNOWLEDGMENTS

The authors would like to acknowledge Yan Li for her help with creating **Figure 2**.

DISCLOSURE

The authors have received research funding from GE Healthcare.

REFERENCES

1. Patel AP, Fisher JL, Nichols E, et al. Global, regional, and national burden of brain and other CNS cancer, 1990–2016: a systematic analysis for the Global Burden of Disease Study 2016. Lancet Neurol 2019;18(4):376–93.
2. Mehta M, Wen P, Nishikawa R, et al. Critical review of the addition of tumor treating fields (TTFields) to the existing standard of care for newly diagnosed glioblastoma patients. Crit Rev Oncol Hematol 2017;111:60–5.
3. Barisano G, Sepehrband F, Ma S, et al. Clinical 7 t MRi: Are we there yet? A review about magnetic resonance imaging at ultra-high field. Br J Radiol 2019;92(1094).
4. Bian W, Hess CP, Chang SM, et al. Susceptibility-weighted MR Imaging of Radiation Therapy-induced Cerebral Microbleeds in Patients with Glioma: A Comparison Between 3T and 7T. Neuroradiology 2014;56(2):91–6.
5. Lupo JM, Li Y, Hess CP, et al. Advances in ultra-high field MRI for the clinical management of patients with brain tumors. Curr Opin Neurol 2011; 24(6):605–15.
6. Springer E, Dymerska B, Cardoso PL, et al. Comparison of Routine Brain Imaging at 3 T and 7 T. Invest Radiol 2016;51(8):469–82.
7. Noebauer-Huhmann IM, Szomolanyi P, Kronnerwetter C, et al. Brain tumours at 7T MRI compared to 3T—contrast effect after half and full standard contrast agent dose: initial results. Eur Radiol 2015;25(1):106–12.
8. Moenninghoff C, Maderwald S, Theysohn JM, et al. Imaging of adult astrocytic brain tumours with 7 T MRI: Preliminary results. Eur Radiol 2010;20(3):704–13.
9. Von Morze C, Xu D, Purcell DD, et al. Intracranial time-of-flight MR angiography at 7T with comparison to 3T. J Magn Reson Imaging 2007;26(4):900–4.
10. Obusez EC, Lowe M, Oh SH, et al. 7T MR of intracranial pathology: Preliminary observations and comparisons to 3T and 1.5T. Neuroimage 2018; 168:459–76.
11. Madai VI, von Samson-Himmelstjerna FC, Bauer M, et al. Ultrahigh-field MRI in human ischemic stroke - a 7 Tesla study. PLoS One 2012;7(5).
12. Tallantyre EC, Morgan PS, Dixon JE, et al. 3 Tesla and 7 Tesla MRI of multiple sclerosis cortical lesions. J Magn Reson Imaging 2010; 32(4):971–7.
13. Schlamann M, Maderwald S, Becker W, et al. Cerebral Cavernous Hemangiomas at 7 Tesla. Initial Experience. Acad Radiol 2010;17(1):3–6.
14. Robitaille PML, Abduljalil AM, Kangarlu A, et al. Human magnetic resonance imaging at 8 T. NMR Biomed 1998;11(6):263–5.
15. Kraff O, Fischer A, Nagel AM, et al. MRI at 7 Tesla and above: Demonstrated and potential capabilities. J Magn Reson Imaging 2015; 41(1):13–33.

16. US Food and Drug Administration (FDA). FDA clears first 7T magnetic resonance imaging device. 2017. Available at: https://www.fda.gov/news-events/press-announcements/fda-clears-first-7t-magnetic-resonance-imaging-device. Accessed May 10, 2020.

17. Artzi M, Bokstein F, Blumenthal DT, et al. Differentiation between vasogenic-edema versus tumor-infiltrative area in patients with glioblastoma during bevacizumab therapy: A longitudinal MRI study. Eur J Radiol 2014;83(7):1250–6.

18. Ginsberg LE, Fuller GN, Hashmi M, et al. The Significance of Lack of MR Contrast Enhancement of Supratentorial Brain Tumors in Adults: Histopathological Evaluation of a Series. Surg Neurol 1998; 49(4):436–40.

19. Bobek-Billewicz B, Stasik-Pres G, Hebda A, et al. Original article Anaplastic transformation of low-grade gliomas (WHO II) on magnetic resonance imaging. Folia Neuropathol 2014;2:128–40.

20. O'Brien KR, Kober T, Hagmann P, et al. Robust T1-weighted structural brain imaging and morphometry at 7T using MP2RAGE. PLoS One 2014;9(6).

21. Jakary A, Hess C, LaFontaine M, et al. Nimg-64. the Potential of 7T Anatomical Imaging for Clinical Assessment of Contrast-Enhancing and T2-Hyperintense Lesions in Patients With Glioma. Neuro Oncol 2017;19(suppl_6):vi156.

22. Christoforidis GA, Grecula JC, Newton HB, et al. Visualization of microvascularity in glioblastoma multiforme with 8-T high-spatial-resolution MR imaging. Am J Neuroradiol 2002;23(9):1553–6.

23. Christoforidis GA, Kangarlu A, Abduljalil AM, et al. Susceptibility-based imaging of glioblastoma microvascularity at 8 T: Correlation of MR imaging and postmortem pathology. Am J Neuroradiol 2004;25(5):756–60.

24. Regnery S, Knowles BR, Paech D, et al. High-resolution FLAIR MRI at 7 Tesla for treatment planning in glioblastoma patients. Radiother Oncol 2019; 130:180–4.

25. Visser F, Zwanenburg JJM, Hoogduin JM, et al. High-resolution magnetization-prepared 3D-FLAIR imaging at 7.0 tesla. Magn Reson Med 2010; 64(1):194–202.

26. van Veluw SJ, Fracasso A, Visser F, et al. FLAIR images at 7 Tesla MRI highlight the ependyma and the outer layers of the cerebral cortex. Neuroimage 2015;104:100–9.

27. Moon HC, Baek H-M, Park YS. Comparison of 3 and 7 Tesla Magnetic Resonance Imaging of Obstructive Hydrocephalus Caused by Tectal Glioma. Brain Tumor Res Treat 2016;4(2):150.

28. Louis DN, Perry A, Reifenberger G, et al. The 2016 World Health Organization Classification of Tumors of the Central Nervous System: a summary. Acta Neuropathol 2016;131(6):1–18.

29. Lev MH, Ozsunar Y, Henson JW, et al. Glial Tumor Grading and Outcome Prediction Using Dynamic Spin-Echo MR Susceptibility Mapping Compared with Conventional Contrast-Enhanced MR: Confounding Effect of Elevated rCBV of Oligodendrogliomas. Am J Neuroradiol 2004;25(2):214–21.

30. Christians A, Adel-Horowski A, Banan R, et al. The prognostic role of IDH mutations in homogeneously treated patients with anaplastic astrocytomas and glioblastomas. Acta Neuropathol Commun 2019; 7(1):156.

31. Yan H, Parsons DW, Jin G, et al. IDH1 and IDH2 Mutations in Gliomas. N Engl J Med 2009;360(8): 765–73.

32. Liu T, Cheng G, Kang X, et al. Noninvasively evaluating the grading and IDH1 mutation status of diffuse gliomas by three-dimensional pseudo-continuous arterial spin labeling and diffusion-weighted imaging. Neuroradiology 2018;60(7): 693–702.

33. Thust SC, Hassanein S, Bisdas S, et al. Apparent diffusion coefficient for molecular subtyping of non-gadolinium-enhancing WHO grade II/III glioma: volumetric segmentation versus two-dimensional region of interest analysis. Eur Radiol 2018;28(9):3779–88.

34. Wu C-C, Jain R, Radmanesh A, et al. Predicting Genotype and Survival in Glioma Using Standard Clinical MR Imaging Apparent Diffusion Coefficient Images: A Pilot Study from The Cancer Genome Atlas. Am J Neuroradiol 2018;39(10): 1814–20.

35. Leu K, Ott GA, Lai A, et al. Perfusion and diffusion MRI signatures in histologic and genetic subtypes of WHO grade II–III diffuse gliomas. J Neurooncol 2017;134(1):177–88.

36. Jenkinson MD, Smith TS, Joyce KA, et al. Cerebral blood volume, genotype and chemosensitivity in oligodendroglial tumours. Neuroradiology 2006; 48(10):703–13.

37. Chawla S, Krejza J, Vossough A, et al. Differentiation between Oligodendroglioma Genotypes Using Dynamic Susceptibility Contrast Perfusion-Weighted Imaging and Proton MR Spectroscopy. Am J Neuroradiol 2013;34(8):1542–9.

38. Tan W, Xiong J, Huang W, et al. Noninvasively detecting Isocitrate dehydrogenase 1 gene status in astrocytoma by dynamic susceptibility contrast MRI. J Magn Reson Imaging 2017; 45(2):492–9.

39. Jalbert LE, Elkhaled A, Phillips JJ, et al. Metabolic Profiling of IDH Mutation and Malignant Progression in Infiltrating Glioma. Sci Rep 2017;7(1):44792.

40. Choi C, Ganji SK, DeBerardinis RJ, et al. 2-hydroxyglutarate detection by magnetic resonance spectroscopy in IDH-mutated patients with gliomas. Nat Med 2012;18(4):624–9.

41. Elkhaled A, Jalbert LE, Phillips JJ, et al. Magnetic Resonance of 2-Hydroxyglutarate in IDH1-Mutated Low-Grade Gliomas. Sci Transl Med 2012;4(116):116ra5.

42. Andronesi OC, Rapalino O, Gerstner E, et al. Detection of oncogenic IDH1 mutations using magnetic resonance spectroscopy of 2-hydroxyglutarate. J Clin Invest 2013;123(9):3659–63.

43. Dang L, White DW, Gross S, et al. Cancer-associated IDH1 mutations produce 2-hydroxyglutarate. Nature 2009;462(7274):739–44.

44. Watanabe T, Nobusawa S, Kleihues P, et al. IDH1 Mutations Are Early Events in the Development of Astrocytomas and Oligodendrogliomas. Am J Pathol 2009;174(4):1149–53.

45. Mohammed W, Xunning H, Haibin S, et al. Clinical applications of susceptibility-weighted imaging in detecting and grading intracranial gliomas: a review. Cancer Imaging 2013;13(2):186–95.

46. Villanueva-Meyer JE, Wood MD, Choi BS, et al. MRI Features and IDH Mutational Status of Grade II Diffuse Gliomas: Impact on Diagnosis and Prognosis. Am J Roentgenol 2018;210(3):621–8.

47. Megyesi JF, Kachur E, Lee DH, et al. Imaging Correlates of Molecular Signatures in Oligodendrogliomas. Clin Cancer Res 2004;10(13):4303–6.

48. Zlatescu MC, TehraniYazdi A, Sasaki H, et al. Tumor location and growth pattern correlate with genetic signature in oligodendroglial neoplasms. Cancer Res 2001;61(18):6713–5. Available at: http://www.ncbi.nlm.nih.gov/pubmed/11559541.

49. Avdievich NI, Pan JW, Baehring JM, et al. Short echo spectroscopic imaging of the human brain at 7T using transceiver arrays. Magn Reson Med 2009;62(1):17–25.

50. Korzowski A, Bachert P. High-resolution 31 P echo-planar spectroscopic imaging in vivo at 7T. Magn Reson Med 2018;79(3):1251–9.

51. Ladd ME, Bachert P, Meyerspeer M, et al. Pros and cons of ultra-high-field MRI/MRS for human application. Prog Nucl Magn Reson Spectrosc 2018;109:1–50.

52. Horská A, Barker P. Imaging of brain tumors: MR spectroscopy and metabolic imaging. Neuroimaging Clin N Am 2010;20(3):293–310.

53. Li Y, Park I, Nelson SJ. Imaging tumor metabolism using in vivo magnetic resonance spectroscopy. Cancer J 2015;21(2):123–8.

54. Tkáč I, Andersen P, Adriany G, et al. In vivo 1 H NMR spectroscopy of the human brain at 7 T. Magn Reson Med 2001;46(3):451–6.

55. Bogner W, Gruber S, Trattnig S, et al. High-resolution mapping of human brain metabolites by free induction decay 1H MRSI at 7 T. NMR Biomed 2012;25(6):873–82.

56. de Graaf RA, Brown PB, McIntyre S, et al. High magnetic field water and metabolite protonT1 andT2 relaxation in rat brain in vivo. Magn Reson Med 2006;56(2):386–94.

57. Otazo R, Mueller B, Ugurbil K, et al. Signal-to-noise ratio and spectral linewidth improvements between 1.5 and 7 Tesla in proton echo-planar spectroscopic imaging. Magn Reson Med 2006;56(6):1200–10.

58. Li Y, Larson P, Chen AP, et al. Short-echo three-dimensional H-1 MR spectroscopic imaging of patients with glioma at 7 tesla for characterization of differences in metabolite levels. J Magn Reson Imaging 2015;41(5):1332–41.

59. Tkáč I, Öz G, Adriany G, et al. In vivo 1 H NMR spectroscopy of the human brain at high magnetic fields: Metabolite quantification at 4T vs. 7T. Magn Reson Med 2009;62(4):868–79.

60. Gruber S, Heckova E, Strasser B, et al. Mapping an Extended Neurochemical Profile at 3 and 7 T Using Accelerated High-Resolution Proton Magnetic Resonance Spectroscopic Imaging. Invest Radiol 2017;52(10):631–9.

61. Henning A, Fuchs A, Murdoch JB, et al. Slice-selective FID acquisition, localized by outer volume suppression (FIDLOVS) for 1 H-MRSI of the human brain at 7 T with minimal signal loss. NMR Biomed 2009;22(7):683–96.

62. Lazovic J, Soto H, Piccioni D, et al. Detection of 2-hydroxyglutaric acid in vivo by proton magnetic resonance spectroscopy in U87 glioma cells overexpressing isocitrate dehydrogenase-1 mutation. Neuro Oncol 2012;14(12):1465–72.

63. Emir E, Larkin S, de Pennington N, et al. The improved detection of 2-hydroxyglutarate in gliomas at 7T using high-bandwidth adiabatic refocusing pulses. In: In Proceedings of the 23rd Annual Meeting of ISMRM. Toronto, Canada, May 30-June 5, 2015. pp. 2236.

64. Ganji S, Hulsey K, Maher EA, et al. In vivo spectroscopic imaging of 2-hydroxyglutarate in human gliomas at 7.0 T. In: In Proceedings of the 21st Annual Meeting of ISMRM. Salt Lake City, UT, April 20-26, 2013. pp. 214.

65. Choi C, Ganji S, Banerjee A, et al. Noninvasive detection of 2-hydroxyglutarate in gliomas by 1H MR spectroscopy at 7.0 T in vivo. In: In Proceedings of the 20th Annual Meeting of ISMRM. Melbourne, Australia, May 5-11, 2012. pp. 1813. 17.

66. Emir UE, Larkin SJ, De Pennington N, et al. Noninvasive quantification of 2-hydroxyglutarate in human gliomas with IDH1 and IDH2 mutations. Cancer Res 2016;76(1):43–9.

67. Ganji SK, An Z, Tiwari V, et al. In vivo detection of 2-hydroxyglutarate in brain tumors by optimized point-resolved spectroscopy (PRESS) at 7T. Magn Reson Med 2017;77(3):936–44.

68. Verma G, Mohan S, Nasrallah MLP, et al. Non-invasive detection of 2-hydroxyglutarate in IDH-mutated gliomas using two-dimensional localized correlation spectroscopy (2D L-COSY) at 7 Tesla. J Transl Med 2016;14(1):1–8.

69. An Z, Tiwari V, Ganji SK, et al. Echo-planar spectroscopic imaging with dual-readout alternated gradients (DRAG-EPSI) at 7 T: Application for 2-hydroxyglutarate imaging in glioma patients. Magn Reson Med 2018;79(4):1851–61.

70. Bisdas S, Chadzynski GL, Braun C, et al. MR spectroscopy for in vivo assessment of the oncometabolite 2-hydroxyglutarate and its effects on cellular metabolism in human brain gliomas at 9.4T. J Magn Reson Imaging 2016;44(4):823–33.

71. Shen X, Voets NL, Larkin SJ, et al. A noninvasive comparison study between human gliomas with IDH1 and IDH2 mutations by MR spectroscopy. Metabolites 2019;9(2):1–11.

72. Moser E, Laistler E, Schmitt F, et al. Ultra-High Field NMR and MRI—The Role of Magnet Technology to Increase Sensitivity and Specificity. Front Physiol 2017;5.

73. Li Y, Lafontaine M, Chang S, et al. Comparison between Short and Long Echo Time Magnetic Resonance Spectroscopic Imaging at 3T and 7T for Evaluating Brain Metabolites in Patients with Glioma. ACS Chem Neurosci 2018;9(1):130–7.

74. Hangel G, Jain S, Springer E, et al. High-resolution metabolic mapping of gliomas via patch-based super-resolution magnetic resonance spectroscopic imaging at 7T. Neuroimage 2019;191:587–95.

75. Mirkes C, Shajan G, Chadzynski G, et al. 31P CSI of the human brain in healthy subjects and tumor patients at 9.4 T with a three-layered multi-nuclear coil: initial results. Magn Reson Mater Phys Biol Med 2016;29(3):579–89.

76. Korzowski A, Weinfurtner N, Mueller S, et al. Volumetric mapping of intra- and extracellular pHl in the human brain using 31P MRSI at 7T. Magn Reson Med 2020;1–17.

77. Ward K, Aletras A, Balaban R. A New Class of Contrast Agents for MRI Based on Proton Chemical Exchange Dependent Saturation Transfer (CEST). J Magn Reson 2000;143(1):79–87.

78. Zhou J, Payen J-F, Wilson DA, et al. Using the amide proton signals of intracellular proteins and peptides to detect pH effects in MRI. Nat Med 2003;9(8):1085–90.

79. Zhou J, Lal B, Wilson DA, et al. Amide proton transfer (APT) contrast for imaging of brain tumors. Magn Reson Med 2003;50(6):1120–6.

80. Sakata A, Okada T, Yamamoto A, et al. Grading glial tumors with amide proton transfer MR imaging: different analytical approaches. J Neurooncol 2015;122(2):339–48.

81. Zhao X, Wen Z, Li C, et al. Quantitative amide proton transfer imaging with reduced interferences from magnetization transfer asymmetry for human brain tumors at 3T. Magn Reson Med 2015;74(1):208–16.

82. Jones CK, Schlosser MJ, van Zijl PCM, et al. Amide proton transfer imaging of human brain tumors at 3T. Magn Reson Med 2006;56(3):585–92.

83. Heo H-Y, Jones CK, Hua J, et al. Whole-brain amide proton transfer (APT) and nuclear overhauser enhancement (NOE) imaging in glioma patients using low-power steady-state pulsed chemical exchange saturation transfer (CEST) imaging at 7T. J Magn Reson Imaging 2016;44(1):41–50.

84. Regnery S, Adeberg S, Dreher C, et al. Chemical exchange saturation transfer MRI serves as predictor of early progression in glioblastoma patients. Oncotarget 2018;9(47):28772–83.

85. Tanoue M, Saito S, Takahashi Y, et al. Amide proton transfer imaging of glioblastoma, neuroblastoma, and breast cancer cells on a 11.7 T magnetic resonance imaging system. Magn Reson Imaging 2019;62:181–90.

86. Paech D, Dreher C, Regnery S, et al. Relaxation-compensated amide proton transfer (APT) MRI signal intensity is associated with survival and progression in high-grade glioma patients. Eur Radiol 2019;29(9):4957–67.

87. Zaiss M, Windschuh J, Goerke S, et al. Downfield-NOE-suppressed amide-CEST-MRI at 7 Tesla provides a unique contrast in human glioblastoma. Magn Reson Med 2017;77(1):196–208.

88. Jones CK, Huang A, Xu J, et al. Nuclear Overhauser enhancement (NOE) imaging in the human brain at 7T. Neuroimage 2013;77(410):114–24.

89. Yao J, Hagiwara A, Raymond C, et al. Human IDH mutant 1p/19q co-deleted gliomas have low tumor acidity as evidenced by molecular MRI and PET: a retrospective study. Sci Rep 2020;10(1):11922.

90. Harris RJ, Cloughesy TF, Liau LM, et al. Simulation, phantom validation, and clinical evaluation of fast pH-weighted molecular imaging using amine chemical exchange saturation transfer echo planar imaging (CEST-EPI) in glioma at 3 T. NMR Biomed 2016;29(11):1563–76.

91. Jones KM, Pollard AC, Pagel MD. Clinical applications of chemical exchange saturation transfer (CEST) MRI. J Magn Reson Imaging 2018;47(1):11–27.

92. Dou W, Lin C-YE, Ding H, et al. Chemical exchange saturation transfer magnetic resonance imaging and its main and potential applications in preclinical and clinical studies. Quant Imaging Med Surg 2019;9(10):1747–66.

93. Neal A, Moffat BA, Stein JM, et al. Glutamate weighted imaging contrast in gliomas with 7 Tesla magnetic resonance imaging. Neuroimage Clin 2019;22:101694.

94. Dreher C, Oberhollenzer J, Meissner JE, et al. Chemical exchange saturation transfer (CEST) signal intensity at 7T MRI of WHO IV° gliomas is dependent on the anatomic location. J Magn Reson Imaging 2019;49(3):777–85.

95. Halefoglu AM, Yousem DM. Susceptibility weighted imaging: Clinical applications and future directions. World J Radiol 2018;10(4):30–45.

96. Rauscher A, Sedlacik J, Barth M, et al. Magnetic susceptibility-weighted MR phase imaging of the human brain. Am J Neuroradiol 2005;26(4):736–42.

97. Hammond KE, Lupo JM, Xu D, et al. Development of a robust method for generating 7.0 T multichannel phase images of the brain with application to normal volunteers and patients with neurological diseases. Neuroimage 2008;39(4):1682–92.

98. Li C, Ai B, Li Y, et al. Susceptibility-weighted imaging in grading brain astrocytomas. Eur J Radiol 2010;75(1):e81–5.

99. Di Ieva A, Göd S, Grabner G, et al. Three-dimensional susceptibility-weighted imaging at 7 T using fractal-based quantitative analysis to grade gliomas. Neuroradiology 2013;55(1):35–40.

100. Grabner G, Kiesel B, Wöhrer A, et al. Local image variance of 7 Tesla SWI is a new technique for preoperative characterization of diffusely infiltrating gliomas: correlation with tumour grade and IDH1 mutational status. Eur Radiol 2017;27(4):1556–67.

101. Lupo JM, Banerjee S, Hammond KE, et al. GRAPPA-based Susceptibility-Weighted Imaging of Normal Volunteers and Patients with Brain Tumor at 7T. Magn Reson Med 2009;27(4):480–8.

102. Biller A, Badde S, Nagel A, et al. Improved brain tumor classification by sodium MR imaging: Prediction of IDH mutation status and tumor progression. Am J Neuroradiol 2016;37(1):66–73.

103. Paech D, Regnery S, Behl N, et al. Sodium MRI at 7 Tesla as quantitative biomarker to assess tumor heterogeneity and histologic subtypes in glioma patients. In: Proceedings of the 28th Annual Meeting of ISMRM. Virtual, 2020. p. 0402.

104. Thulborn KR. Quantitative sodium MR imaging: A review of its evolving role in medicine. Neuroimage 2018;168:250–68.

105. Wu Y, Agarwal S, Jones CK, et al. Measurement of arteriolar blood volume in brain tumors using MRI without exogenous contrast agent administration at 7T. J Magn Reson Imaging 2016;44(5):1244–55.

106. Jackson A. Magnetic resonance perfusion imaging in neuro-oncology. Cancer Imaging 2008;8(1):186–99.

107. Law M, Yang S, Babb JS, et al. Comparison of cerebral blood volume and vascular permeability from dynamic susceptibility contrast-enhanced perfusion MR imaging with glioma grade. Am J Neuroradiol 2004;25(5):746–55.

108. Cha S, Tihan T, Crawford F, et al. Differentiation of low-grade oligodendrogliomas from low-grade astrocytomas by using quantitative blood-volume measurements derived from dynamic susceptibility contrast-enhanced MR imaging. Am J Neuroradiol 2005;26(2):266–73.

109. Law M, Young R, Babb J, et al. Histogram analysis versus region of interest analysis of dynamic susceptibility contrast perfusion MR imaging data in the grading of cerebral gliomas. Am J Neuroradiol 2007;28(4):761–6.

110. Rutland JW, Delman BN, Gill CM, et al. Emerging use of ultra-high-field 7T MRI in the study of intracranial vascularity: State of the field and future directions. Am J Neuroradiol 2020;41(1):2–9.

111. Thorsen F, Fite B, Mahakian LM, et al. Multimodal imaging enables early detection and characterization of changes in tumor permeability of brain metastases. J Control Release 2013;172(3):812–22.

112. Mönninghoff C, Maderwald S, Theysohn J, et al. Imaging of Brain Metastases of Bronchial Carcinomas with 7 T MRI – Initial Results. RöFo 2010;182(09):764–72.

113. Eichler AF, Chung E, Kodack DP, et al. The biology of brain metastases—translation to new therapies. Nat Rev Clin Oncol 2011;8(6):344–56.

114. Nieman LK. Recent Updates on the Diagnosis and Management of Cushing's Syndrome. Endocrinol Metab 2018;33(2):139.

115. Law M, Wang R, Liu CSJ, et al. Value of pituitary gland MRI at 7 T in Cushing's disease and relationship to inferior petrosal sinus sampling: Case report. J Neurosurg 2019;130(2):347–51.

116. de Rotte AAJ, Groenewegen A, Rutgers DR, et al. High resolution pituitary gland MRI at 7.0 tesla: a clinical evaluation in Cushing's disease. Eur Radiol 2016;26(1):271–7.

117. Van Der Kolk AG, Hendrikse J, Zwanenburg JJM, et al. Clinical applications of 7 T MRI in the brain. Eur J Radiol 2013;82(5):708–18.

118. Sanai N, Berger MS. Operative techniques for gliomas and the value of extent of resection. Neurotherapeutics 2009;6(3):478–86.

119. Kekhia H, Rigolo L, Norton I, et al. Special surgical considerations for functional brain mapping. Neurosurg Clin N Am 2011;22(2):111–32.

120. Morrison MA, Churchill NW, Cusimano MD. Reliability of Task-Based fMRI for Preoperative Planning: A Test-Retest Study in Brain Tumor Patients and Healthy Controls. PLoS One 2016;1–25.

121. Morrison MA, Tam F, Garavaglia MM, et al. Sources of Variation Influencing Concordance between Functional MRI and Direct Cortical

Stimulation in Brain Tumor Surgery. Front Neurosci 2016;10:461.

122. Trattnig S, Springer E, Bogner W, et al. Key clinical benefits of neuroimaging at 7 T Europe PMC Funders Group. Neuroimage 2018;168:477–89.

123. Triantafyllou C, Hoge RD, Krueger G, et al. Comparison of physiological noise at 1.5 T, 3 T and 7 T and optimization of fMRI acquisition parameters. Neuroimage 2005;26(1):243–50.

124. Duong TQ, Yacoub E, Adriany G, et al. Microvascular BOLD contribution at 4 and 7 T in the human brain: Gradient-echo and spin-echo fMRI with suppression of blood effects. Magn Reson Med 2003; 49(6):1019–27.

125. van der Zwaag W, Francis S, Head K, et al. fMRI at 1.5, 3 and 7 T: Characterising BOLD signal changes. Neuroimage 2009;47(4):1425–34.

126. Gizewski ER, de Greiff A, Maderwald S, et al. fMRI at 7 T: Whole-brain coverage and signal advantages even infratentorially? Neuroimage 2007; 37(3):761–8.

127. Beisteiner R, Robinson S, Wurnig M, et al. Clinical fMRI: Evidence for a 7T benefit over 3T. Neuroimage 2011;57(3):1015–21.

128. Lima Cardoso P, Dymerska B, Bachratá B, et al. The clinical relevance of distortion correction in presurgical fMRI at 7 T. Neuroimage 2018;168: 490–8.

129. Wen Q, Kelley DAC, Banerjee S, et al. Clinically feasible NODDI characterization of glioma using multiband EPI at 7 T. Neuroimage Clin 2015;9: 291–9.

130. Peerlings J, Compter I, Janssen F, et al. Characterizing geometrical accuracy in clinically optimised 7T and 3T magnetic resonance images for high-precision radiation treatment of brain tumours. Phys Imaging Radiat Oncol 2019;9:35–42.

131. Eekers DB, In 't Ven L, Roelofs E, et al. The EPTN consensus based atlas for CT- and MR-based contouring in neuro-oncology. Radiother Oncol 2018; 128(1):37–43.

132. Grabner G, Nöbauer I, Elandt K, et al. Longitudinal brain imaging of five malignant glioma patients treated with bevacizumab using susceptibility-weighted magnetic resonance imaging at 7 T. Magn Reson Imaging 2012;30(1): 139–47.

133. Lupo JM, Essock-Burns E, Molinaro AM, et al. Using susceptibility-weighted imaging to determine response to combined antiangiogenic, cytotoxic, and radiation therapy in patients with glioblastoma multiforme. Neuro Oncol 2013; 15(4):480–9.

134. Meissner J, Korzowski A, Regnery S, et al. Early response assessment of glioma patients to definitive chemoradiotherapy using chemical exchange

saturation transfer imaging at 7 T. J Magn Reson Imaging 2019;50(4):1268–77.

135. Huang L, Zhang Z, Qu B, et al. Imaging of Sodium MRI for Therapy Evaluation of Brain Metastase with Cyberknife at 7T: A Case Report. Cureus 2018; 10(4).

136. Srinivasan R, Phillips JJ, Berg SRV, et al. Ex vivo MR spectroscopic measure differentiates tumor from treatment effects in GBM. Neuro Oncol 2010;12(11):1152–61.

137. Castillo M, Smith JK, Kwock L. Correlation of myoinositol levels and grading of cerebral astrocytomas. Am J Neuroradiol 2000;21(9):1645–9.

138. Lupo JM, Chuang C, Chang SM, et al. 7 Tesla Susceptibility-Weighted Imaging to Assess the Effects of Radiation Therapy on Normal Appearing Brain in Patients with Glioma. Int J Radiat Oncol Biol Phys 2012;82(2):493–500.

139. Conijn MMA, Geerlings MI, Biessels GJ, et al. Cerebral microbleeds on MR imaging: Comparison between 1.5 and 7T. Am J Neuroradiol 2011; 32(6):1043–9.

140. Kuijf HJ, de Bresser J, Geerlings MI, et al. Efficient detection of cerebral microbleeds on 7.0T MR images using the radial symmetry transform. Neuroimage 2012;59(3):2266–73.

141. Bian W, Hess CP, Chang SM, et al. Computer-aided detection of radiation-induced cerebral microbleeds on susceptibility-weighted MR images. Neuroimage Clin 2013;2(1):282–90.

142. Morrison MA, Payabvash S, Chen Y, et al. A user-guided tool for semi-automated cerebral microbleed detection and volume segmentation: Evaluating vascular injury and data labelling for machine learning. Neuroimage Clin 2018;20: 498–505.

143. Chen Y, Villanueva-Meyer JE, Morrison MA, et al. Toward Automatic Detection of Radiation-Induced Cerebral Microbleeds Using a 3D Deep Residual Network. J Digit Imaging 2019;32(5):766–72.

144. Morrison MA, Hess CP, Clarke JL, et al. Risk factors of radiotherapy-induced cerebral microbleeds and serial analysis of their size compared with white matter changes: A 7T MRI study in 113 adult patients with brain tumors. J Magn Reson Imaging 2019;50(3):868–77.

145. Lupo JM, Molinaro AM, Essock-Burns E, et al. The effects of anti-angiogenic therapy on the formation of radiation-induced microbleeds in normal brain tissue of patients with glioma. Neuro Oncol 2016; 18(1):87–95.

146. Theysohn JM, Kraff O, Maderwald S, et al. 7 Tesla MRI of microbleeds and white matter lesions as seen in vascular dementia. J Magn Reson Imaging 2011;33(4):782–91.

147. Bian W, Banerjee S, Kelly DAC, et al. Simultaneous imaging of radiation-induced cerebral microbleeds,

arteries and veins, using a multiple gradient echo sequence at 7 Tesla. J Magn Reson Imaging 2015; 42(2):269–79.

148. De Bresser J, Brundel M, Conijn MM, et al. Visual cerebral microbleed detection on 7T MR imaging: Reliability and effects of image processing. Am J Neuroradiol 2013;34(6).

149. Conijn MMA, Geerlings MI, Luijten PR, et al. Visualization of cerebral microbleeds with dual-echo T2*-weighted magnetic resonance imaging at 7.0 T. J Magn Reson Imaging 2010;32(1):52–9.

150. Wahl M, Anwar M, Hess CP, et al. Relationship between radiation dose and microbleed formation in patients with malignant glioma. Radiat Oncol 2017;12(1):126.

151. Belliveau J-G, Bauman GS, Tay KY, et al. Initial Investigation into Microbleeds and White Matter Signal Changes following Radiotherapy for Low-Grade and Benign Brain Tumors Using Ultra-High-Field MRI Techniques. Am J Neuroradiol 2017;38(12):2251–6.

152. Morrison M, Avadiappan S, Yuan J, et al. NIMG-56. A multimodal 7 Telsa MRI investigation of long-term effects of radiotherapy on the adolescent brain & cognition. Neuro Oncol 2019;21(Supplement_6): vi173–4.

153. Avadiappan S, Morrison M, Jakary A, et al. RTHP-21. Characterization of radiation therapy effects on cerebral vasculature in pediatric brain tumor survivors. Neuro Oncol 2018;20(suppl_6):vi229.

MR-EYE: High-Resolution MRI of the Human Eye and Orbit at Ultrahigh Field (7T)

Rebecca K. Glarin, PGDipMRI[a,b,*], Bao N. Nguyen, PhD[c],
Jon O. Cleary, MD, PhD[a,d], Scott C. Kolbe, PhD[e], Roger J. Ordidge, PhD[a],
Bang V. Bui, PhD[c], Allison M. McKendrick, PhD[c], Bradford A. Moffat, PhD[a]

KEYWORDS

• MRI • 7T • Ultrahigh field • Eye • Ophthalmic imaging • Myopia • Presbyopia • Glaucoma

KEY POINTS

- Dedicated eye imaging can be implemented at 7T to acquire high-resolution, high contrast-to-noise, and high signal-to-noise images in a feasible imaging time suitable for clinical use.
- Simple, reproducible participant preparation techniques can be adopted to reduce the motion of the eye leading to a reduction in subsequent artefacts.
- Sequences available at ultrahigh field can be used in current 7T clinical applications to visualize ocular structures otherwise impossible with other ophthalmic imaging.

 Video content accompanies this article at http://www.mri.theclinics.com.

INTRODUCTION

The adult eye is approximately 2.3 cm in length, comprising tissue structures that are often less than a millimeter in size. Clinically, posterior eye imaging of the retina is frequently conducted using optical coherence tomography (OCT), which uses low-coherence interferometry of light to determine the relative depth of structures. OCT only enables imaging of biological tissues within approximately a millimeter of the surface, however, because light can penetrate the eye through the pupil to reach the retina; the technique enables imaging of retinal structures at the posterior eye. Compared with MRI, OCT has a better axial resolution ($\sim$3.5 µm) and allows visualization of the distinct retinal layers

and the underlying vascular choroid (chor). However, the lateral field of view is limited (typically <1 cm of the retina is imaged at a time, although newer wide-field imaging exists), and there is limited penetration (approximately 1–1.5 mm) into the retina (**Fig. 1A, B**). Furthermore, for eyes that are abnormally elongated (such as highly myopic eyes that tend to have a steepening of the retina posteriorly[1]), the OCT-displayed retinal curvature does not readily represent true anatomy as the device algorithm artificially flattens the 2D OCT image.[2]

On the other hand, MRI can noninvasively image the entire eyeball, orbit, and retrobulbar structures, without optical distortion[3] (**Fig. 1C**). For some time now, high-field MRI has been used to

[a] The Melbourne Brain Centre Imaging Unit, Department of Medicine and Radiology, The University of Melbourne, Parkville, Victoria 3010, Australia; [b] Department of Radiology, Royal Melbourne Hospital, Parkville, Victoria 3010, Australia; [c] Department of Optometry and Vision Sciences, The University of Melbourne, Parkville, Victoria 3010, Australia; [d] Department of Radiology, Guy's and St. Thomas' NHS Foundation Trust, Westminster Bridge Road, London SE1 7EH, UK; [e] Department of Neuroscience, Central Clinical School, Monash University, Prahran, Victoria 3181, Australia
* Corresponding author. Melbourne Brain Centre Imaging Unit, Department of Radiology, The University of Melbourne, Kenneth Myer Building, Parkville, Victoria 3010, Australia.
E-mail address: rebecca.glarin@unimelb.edu.au

Magn Reson Imaging Clin N Am 29 (2021) 103–116
https://doi.org/10.1016/j.mric.2020.09.004

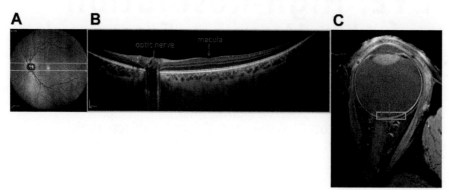

Fig. 1. (*A*) En-face image of the posterior eye (ocular fundus) showing the horizontal position of the optic nerve and macula (*red arrows*, corresponding to labels in panel B). The green box indicates the field of view currently possible with a wide-field lens (enabling 55° diameter view) and optical coherence. (*B*) An example of wide-field OCT b-scan showing the axial resolution of OCT in distinguishing the retinal layers and underlying vascular choroid. The horizontal position of the optic nerve and macula (*red arrows*) are labeled. (*C*) A 3D gradient-echo MRI image of the eye (TR/TE = 10/4 ms, 0.2 × 0.2 × 0.4 mm resolution) with superimposed green box as a schematic to indicate the maximum field of view currently possible with OCT compared with the whole eye/orbit imaging possible with MRI.

investigate the etiology of cataract[4] and presbyopia,[5] albeit *in vitro*. With increased whole-body MRI field strengths and the development of small-surface radiofrequency (RF) coils,[6,7] it has become possible to visualize and study the whole eye *in vivo*. As such, applications have expanded to studying other ocular conditions such as myopia, glaucoma, and intraocular tumors.[8,9] Accordingly, clinical MRI referrals to image the eye and orbit for diagnosis and management of ocular masses are ever-increasing, although such imaging can be hampered by the image resolution, and motion and susceptibility artifacts.[10]

For the most part, clinical MRI of the eye and surrounding orbit has been conducted with a head coil or orbital coil at conventional field strengths (3T or 1.5 T).[11,12] The increase in signal-to-noise ratio (SNR) at 7T compared with conventional clinical scanners of 1.5 T and 3T[13] has allowed for a discussion[14] on the implementation of 7T imaging to benefit neuro-ophthalmology work. Here, we describe the use of a dedicated commercial multichannel eye coil at ultrahigh-field (7 T) magnetic field strength to acquire 2D and 3D images of ocular anatomy. With careful consideration of participant preparation and sequence selection to maximize the image quality, the first aim of this study was to demonstrate clinically feasible ultrahigh-field ocular and orbital MRI with minimal motion[14] and susceptibility artifacts. The hypothesis was that the phased array eye coil would offer the ability to reduce the scanning times of high-resolution and high-contrast[15] sequences such that a very simple fixation setup would be sufficient and successful to reduce artifact from the

eye movement and position. Furthermore, we aimed to remove the need for more time-intensive techniques such as blink detection to remove motion artifacts,[16,17] in order to assist high-resolution MRI to be transferred into a clinical setting. The second study aim was to demonstrate the application of these techniques for quantitative studies of the ocular tissue dimension and shape, retrobulbar ocular anatomy, and the effect of gaze on the optic nerve.[11,18] In order to address the hypothesis, it was necessary to assess the image quality through the region of interest (ROI) calculations and MRI parameter investigations along with reproducibility of the image quality. Our findings can be used to improve MRI investigations of an array of ocular conditions such as myopia, glaucoma, ocular tumors, cataract, and presbyopia.[9]

METHODS
Apparatus and Safety Assessment

The study protocol was approved by the Human Research Ethics Committee at The University of Melbourne (ID 1646275 and 1340926). Participants provided written informed consent before imaging. In total, 11 healthy participants (aged 20–41 years) free of ocular pathology were recruited. They were emmetropic, with spherical refractive errors between −0.50D and +0.75D, with normal visual acuity (6/7.5 or better) and normal ocular health as determined by a screening eye examination (BNN).

We performed ultrahigh-field MRI using a 7 T whole-body scanner (Magnetom, Siemens

Healthcare, Erlangen, Germany) and a six-element transmit/receive RF eye coil (MRI.TOOLS GmbH, Berlin, Germany), which is based on a prototype published by Graessl and colleagues[15] 2013 (**Fig. 2**). The RF coil has a symmetric design with six overlapping 36-mm diameter transceiver loop elements tuned to 297 MHz. A custom-built coil holder was fabricated from Perspex plastic to assist with coil placement (see **Fig. 2**A). The aim of the holder design was to enable coil stabilization and participant comfort and to minimize the distance from the skin to the eye coil without any skin contact. The design included the need to have the ability of height adjustment to accommodate for differing participant head shapes. Positioning the coil as close to the eye as possible allowed for maximum posterior eye anatomy to be visible without any hindrance from the signal loss related to the use of a surface coil.[6,14,15] Scanning was conducted at the Melbourne Brain Centre Imaging Unit (Parkville, VIC, Australia) for no more than 1 hour. All participants were screened by the radiographer to ensure they were safe to be scanned.

Participant Preparation

There are inherent problems associated with imaging the eye *in vivo*, the most common being motion artifacts caused by the involuntary eye movements (microsaccades) that occur several times per second.[14] Although the gain in the SNR of ultrahigh-field MRI would be beneficial for imaging the small structures of the eye, based on previous 7T studies,[14,15] it was expected that susceptibility artifacts would also increase significantly with increasing field strength. Hence, it is critical that patients are prepared well to optimize imaging, and we were careful to follow previous suggestions for participant preparation.[8,14,17,19]

such as taping the eyelid of the imaged eye shut to prevent blinking and reduce susceptibility artifacts from the air-tissue interface (**Fig. 3**A vs 3B).

In addition, we developed our own fixation technique to maximize participant stability (**Fig. 3**C vs 3D). With one eye taped shut (the eye to be imaged), the other was allowed to fixate. Under normal circumstances, the eyes are yoked and will move together. Thus, if the fixating eye stays still, so too will the imaged eye. The participant was asked to look into the mirror attached to the coil that showed the fixation target on an LCD screen positioned at the far end of the magnet bore. With proper placement of the target cross on the screen, so that the fixating eye could view the fixation target centrally (hence the fixation target was shifted laterally from the center of view according to each person's individual interpupillary distance, ~12° of visual angle), a comfortable neutral eye position could be maintained without strain and movement. To maintain attention, the participant was given a button box and asked to press a button whenever the fixation target changed color (Video 1). Furthermore, given the potential for dry eye within the scanner from the fans, as well as from a reduced blink rate due to concentration, we found that instillation of ocular lubricants (TheraTears, Akorn Consumer Health, Ann Arbor, MI, USA) before scanning assisted in participant comfort.

SEQUENCE CHOICE AND CONSIDERATIONS FOR OPTIMIZATION TO VISUALIZE RELEVANT ANATOMY

Our aim of acquiring data with a high SNR and contrast-to-noise ratio (CNR) required the optimization of essential imaging factors for clinical use. We addressed these in the following subexperiments:

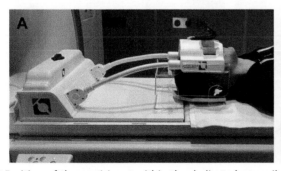
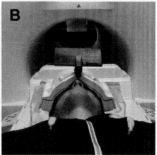

Fig. 2. (*A*) Position of the participant within the dedicated eye coil (sagittal view). The eye coil was a 6-channel transmit/receive eye coil array (297 MHz, icoil, MRI.TOOLS GmbH, Berlin, Germany). The custom-built coil holder could be adjusted to the optimal height for each participant. (*B*) The position of the participant within the dedicated eye coil (transverse view).

- Experiment one—flip angle assessment in 3D gradient echo (GRE) imaging;
- Experiment two—increase in resolution of 3D GRE imaging;
- Experiment three—echo time assessment in 3D GRE imaging;
- Experiment four—reproducibility of the SNR and CNR in 3D GRE imaging;
- Experiment five—Visualization of the optic nerve thickness in coronal T2 turbo spin echo (TSE);
- Experiment six—echo time assessment and visualization of the optic nerve position in axial T2 TSE.

3D Gradient-Echo Imaging—Fast Low-Angle Snapshot T1-Weighted MRI

High-resolution true 3D MRI data can be acquired using an RF spoiled 3D FLASH sequence. The axial orbital length (the distance from the anterior surface of the cornea and the central fovea of the retina) can be measured, and all ocular tissues from the cornea through to the optic tract are demonstrated.[8,15] Consideration was required to optimize the sequence CNR and SNR to visualize these structures.

Experiment one was a GRE sequence with fat saturation, acquired for one eye in the axial plane aimed at optimizing flip-angle allocation. The

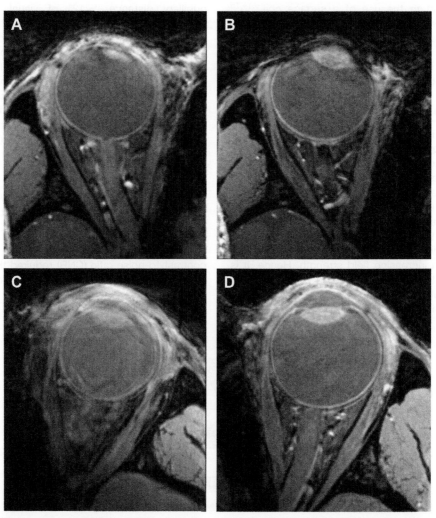

Fig. 3. 3D GRE axial images (TR/TE = 13/4 ms, FA = 12°, 0.2 × 0.2 × 0.9 mm resolution) of the eye demonstrating differing patient preparation: (A) the eye shut but not taped, (B) the eye open, producing susceptibility artifact, (C) the eye taped and closed, no fixation task with the opposing eye (motion artifact), and (D) with our fixation task showing very little artifact.

participant had the chosen eye imaged 6 times. The acquisition was a 2′24″ second acquisition repeated 6 times with varied excitation flip angles (5, 10, 12, 15, 20, and 30°) to determine the optimal contrast for visualization of the main ocular tissues (**Fig. 4**). Imaging parameters for the GRE sequence were a repetition time/echo time (TR/TE) = 13/4 ms, in-plane 81-mm field of view (FOV), voxel dimensions of 0.2 × 0.2 × 0.9 mm, flip angle (FA) = 12, matrix size of 384 x 384 pixels, 44 slices and a GRAPPA acceleration factor of 2.

Experiment two consisted of a 4-min, higher resolution version of the GRE at an optimized flip angle of 12° derived from the previous experiment. All parameters were the same as the first experiment, except the slice resolution was 0.4 mm and TR was 10 ms (**Fig. 5**A, B). The aim was to increase the resolution as far as possible while maintaining an achievable scan time.

Experiment three was a TE investigation with respect to optic nerve evaluation. The same GRE sequence was used as in experiment

two: 0.2 x 0.2 x 0.4 resolution and repeated with a TE of 4 ms and 10 ms (**Fig. 6**).

Experiment four was a reproducibility study of the SNR, CNR, and artifacts of 11 healthy emmetropic participants using the parameters from experiment one with an optimized flip angle of 12°, derived from experiment one (**Fig. 7**).

Coronal Oblique T2 Measurements of Retrobulbar Ocular Anatomy

A significant advantage of MRI is the ability to visualize structures behind the eyeball *in vivo*. We exploited this fact and conducted T2-weighted measurements of retrobulbar ocular anatomy. After the optic nerve exits the eyeball, it becomes myelinated and as it travels posteriorly to the optic chiasm, the optic nerve is surrounded by a subarachnoid space (ss) (filled with fluid, contiguous with cerebrospinal fluid), which is surrounded by the optic nerve sheath (ons) (membrane). We aimed to use ultrahigh-field MRI with slices less than 1 mm to minimize partial volume artifact to

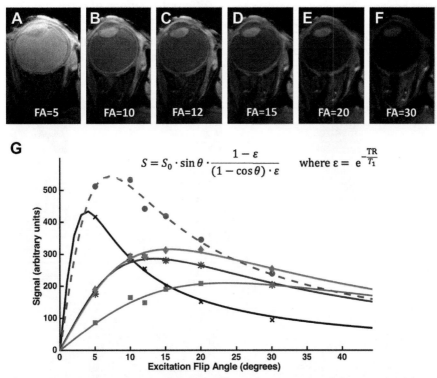

Fig. 4. Multiflip angle experiment data. (*A–F*) Images of 2 representative axial slices acquired from a GRE with varied flip angles (FA or θ) of 5, 10, 12, 15, 20, and 30°. TR/TE = 13/4 ms, 0.2 × 0.2 × 0.9 mm. (*G*) The MRI signal (arbitrary units) as a function of the flip angle from the lens (red circle), vitreous (*blue cross*), optic nerve (*000*), lateral muscle (*purple star*), and fatty tissue (*light blue square*). Lines represent nonlinear least square fitting to a well-known nuclear magnetic resonance equation.

Equation in figure:
$$S = S_0 \cdot \sin\theta \cdot \frac{1-\varepsilon}{(1-\cos\theta)\cdot\varepsilon} \quad \text{where } \varepsilon = e^{-\frac{TR}{T_1}}$$

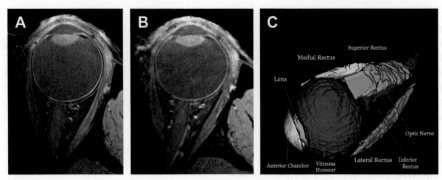

Fig. 5. GRE = TR/TE 10/4, in-plane 81-mm FOV, FA = 12, matrix size of 384 x 384 pixels, 44 slices, and a GRAPPA acceleration factor of 2. (*A*) Voxel dimensions of 0.2 × 0.2 × 0.4 mm, acquisition time 4:26 minutes, (*B*) voxel dimensions of 0.2 × 0.2 × 0.9 mm, acquisition time 2:24 minutes, and (*C*) semi-automated segmentation and 3D rendering of those in panel A, performed with the ITK-Snap toolbox.

enable more accurate demarcation of the retrobulbar optic nerve and its surrounding anatomy.[20,21]

In experiment five, we conducted 2D coronal oblique cross-sectional scans (TR/TE = 2000/64 ms, in-plane 155 mm FOV, voxel dimensions of 0.4 × 0.4 × 0.7 mm, matrix = 384 x 384 pixels, 14 slices (7 each eye), scan time = 2′34" (**Fig. 8A–D**)) on all 11 participants. The slices were angled perpendicular to each individual's optic nerve with these slice positions allocated according to an initial 2D T2-weighted fast spin echo axial planning scan without fat suppression (TR/TE = 2130/73 ms, FOV = 150 mm, voxel dimensions = 0.4 ×

0.4 × 0.7 mm, matrix = 384 x 384 pixels, 12 slice, scan time = 2′06") (**Fig. 8E**). The acquisitions were optimized to acquire both optic nerves in the same acquisition using 2 slice groups. It is important to consider the signal void from crosstalk if the two groups intercept close to the optic nerve.

Axial Oblique T2 Measurements of the Different Positions of Gaze and Created Tension on the Optic Nerve

High-resolution orbital MRI has recreated interest in using the technology in conjunction with gaze

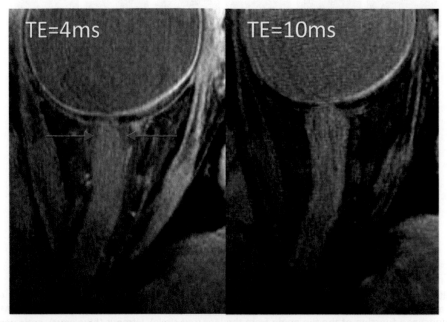

Fig. 6. GRE with varied TE of 4 and 10 ms, all other parameters set as TR = 13, in-plane 81-mm FOV, voxel dimensions of 0.2 × 0.2 × 0.9 mm, FA = 12, matrix size of 384 x 384 pixels, 44 slices, and a GRAPPA acceleration factor of 2. Note clearer delineation of the optic nerve borders on the TE = 4 ms (*red arrows*).

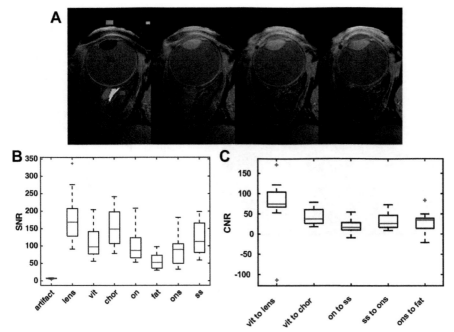

Fig. 7. (*A*) Four central slices from an example set of 3D GRE axial images (TR/TE = 13/4 ms, FA = 12°, 2 × 0.2 × 0.9 mm resolution) of the eye and orbit. For optimal image quality, the imaged eye is taped shut while the participant fixates on a flashing target with the contralateral eye. (*B, C*) Box plots displaying the distribution of SNR and CNR across various orbit tissues in 11 healthy, emmetropic participants, respectively. Tissue ROIs are shown as color patches: lens (*blue*), vitreous humor (vit, *dark purple*), choroid (chor, *red*), optic nerve (on, *dark green*), subarachnoid space (ss, *cyan*), optic nerve sheath (ons, *yellow*), retro-orbital fat (fat, *light purple*), artifact (*orange*), and noise (*light green*). The central mark is the median, the edges of the box are the 25th and 75th percentiles, the whiskers extend to the most extreme data points the algorithm considers to be not outliers, and the outliers are plotted individually.

and the ability to contribute to the investigation of mechanical forces on the optic nerve.[2,22]

In experiment six, we demonstrate the use of ultrahigh-field MRI to image the eye and its optic nerve during horizontal duction (left or right gaze, **Fig. 9**), relative to a neutral position using 2D T2-weighted fast spin echo axial scans without fat suppression (TR/TE = 2130/73 ms, FOV = 150 mm, voxel dimensions = 0.4 × 0.4 × 0.7 mm, matrix = 384 x 384 pixels, 12 slice, scan time = 2′06″). Initially, a single subject was scanned at varying echo times of 27, 45, and 73 ms (**Fig. 10**). Then, from 11 healthy emmetropic participants, data were acquired using the optimized protocol (TE = 45 ms without fat sat at 7T).

Statistics

The SNR and CNR were quantified for ROIs (see **Fig. 7**A) from 11 emmetropes. The ROIs, shown in **Fig. 7**A, were drawn manually, by an MRI scientist (BAM) with substantial experience applying MRI to vision science, using MATLAB (Natick, MA, USA). The mean and standard deviations of variations of the SNR and CNR were then

calculated; the SNR being defined as the ratio of image intensity to standard deviation of voxel intensities from air and the CNR being defined as the difference in the SNR from adjacent tissues.

RESULTS AND DISCUSSION

Experiments 1 to 4: T1-Weighted GRE FLASH MRI

Ipsilateral eye closed and contralateral eye fixated is the optimal participant setup

As with previous studies, GRE FLASH images are much improved when the imaged eye is closed (see **Fig. 3**D).[6,14,15,21] When the eye is open (see **Fig. 3**B), the magnetic susceptibility difference between the air and cornea creates severe magnetic field inhomogeneities leading to signal heterogeneity caused by decreased T2* relaxation times. This inhomogeneity extends beyond the lens and into the vitreous when the eye is left open. Although advanced automatic and manual shimming strategies including shim volume placement were explored, these proved to make little difference possibly because of the involuntary eye movement. Although in theory we expected

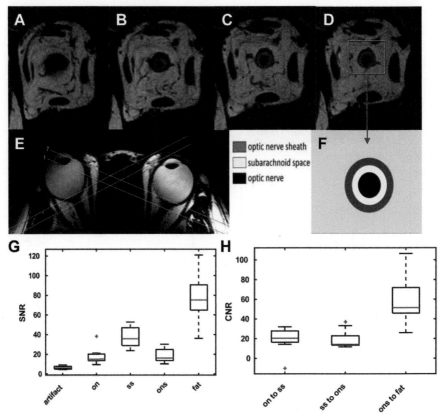

Fig. 8. (*A–D*) Coronal oblique slices through the optic nerve starting from the insertion point (*A*), with anatomic regions of interest available for identification and quantification if required in panel F. (*E*) Slice locations of the coronal oblique images in panels A to D representing slice 4, 3, 2, and 1 of the right eye. Sequence parameters for the coronal oblique—TR/TE = 2000/64 ms, voxel dimensions of 0.4 × 0.4 × 0.7 mm, 14 slices, 7 on each optic nerve. Slice locations demonstrated manually using in-built tools in biomedical imaging software. (*G*, *H*) Box plot showing SNR and CNR distributions from 11 healthy emmetropic participants, respectively. The central mark is the median, the edges of the box are the 25th and 75th percentiles, the whiskers extend to the most extreme data points the algorithm considers to be not outliers, and the outliers are plotted individually.

shorter scan durations would improve imaging, this was not as problematic as initially thought. We found that even with a scan duration of 2 to 2.5 minutes, severe motion artifacts (see **Fig. 3**C) occurred when the participant was not asked to fixate using an interactive task. However, with fixation on a customized and interactive task (see **Fig. 3**D), these artifacts were dramatically reduced.

Turn off unnecessary coil elements during reception

An important consideration was coil application. During acquisition, only the 3 receiver loops over the eye of interest were activated, reducing motion artifact from the other eye.[15] For illustrative purpose, **Fig. 11** displays the signal from the 6 individual coil elements. By eliminating the coils with limited signal but noticeable motion artifact, this

will benefit the resultant image. This selective coil method also limited the amount of signal from outside the field of view being available for reconstruction and causing a wrap artifact in the displayed image.[15]

Optimize contrast by matching excitation the flip angle to ocular tissues of interest

In experiment one by varying the flip angle (see **Fig. 4**) of these 3D FLASH images, it can be seen that the signal and contrast of the images can be controlled to optimize the data depending on which particular ocular tissue is of interest. By inspecting the change in the various tissue signals with the flip angle (see **Fig. 4**G), we determined that a nominal flip angle of 12° produced a good compromise of signal and contrast for visualization of the lens, vitreous, retina, and optic nerve.

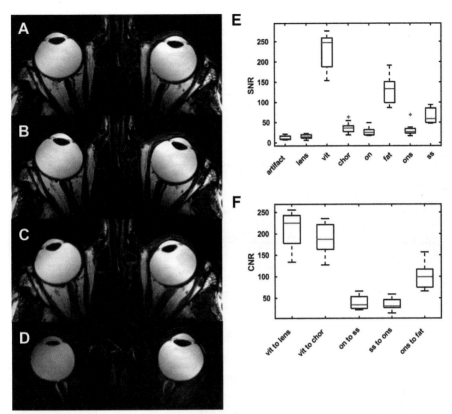

Fig. 9. Axial oblique T2-weighted images aligned with the optic nerve in 3 gaze positions: neutral gaze (*A*), left gaze (*B*), and right gaze (*C*). Imaging parameters (*A–C*): TR/TE = 2130/73 ms, voxel dimensions = 0.4 × 0.4 × 0.7 mm. Axial T2 image with fat saturation in the neutral gaze position is also shown (*D*). Note the enhancement of CSF surrounding the optic nerve but the loss of the signal from other anatomic structures. (*E, F*) A box plot of SNR and CNR distributions of various orbit tissues within 11 healthy emmetropic participants. The central mark is the median, the edges of the box are the 25th and 75th percentiles, the whiskers extend to the most extreme data points the algorithm considers to be not outliers, and the outliers are plotted individually.

3D GRE achieves the highest possible image resolution

In experiments two and three, while assessing the resolution and TE of the 3D GRE, on a single participant, a 4-min higher resolution (0.2 × 0.2 × 0.4 mm voxels) was achievable with minimal artifact (see **Fig. 5**A). The high-resolution images in experiment two displayed the depth of structure identification possible to have positive results for segmentation of anatomy. The marked borders of the globe itself allows for volumetric measurements and 3D modeling (see **Fig. 5**C).

Minimum TE provides optimal contrast and minimized artifacts

The results of experiment three (see **Fig. 6**) indicate that extending the echo time substantially decreases the contrast and signal, while also increasing T2*-related susceptibility with artifacts easily seen on structure borders such as extraocular muscles. There was a clear visual difference in

the borders of the optic nerve (see **Fig. 6**) when the minimum TE was used. This definition is vital for further studies where we aim to assess the optic nerve in more detail.

Resolution is limited by participant compliance

Subjectively through experiments one, two, and three, it was concluded that not all participants or future clinical cohorts would be able to complete the high-resolution scanning without motion artifacts despite fixation tasks. These observations meant the reproducibility study (experiment four) would be more successful with utilization of the 2′, 0.4 x 0.4 x 0.9 resolution protocol.

3D GRE imaging provides visualization of all the major tissues in the orbit with a reproducibly excellent SNR and CNR

The results of experiment 4 are shown as boxplots in **Fig. 7**B, C. The SNR results of the lens, vitreous humor, choroid, optic nerve, subarachnoid space,

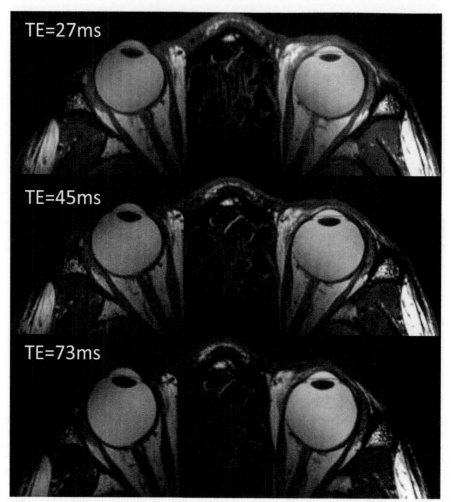

Fig. 10. Axial T2 with varied TE of 27, 45 and 73 ms on a healthy 26-year-old man. Other imaging parameters: TR = 2130 ms, FOV = 150 mm, voxel dimensions = 0.4 × 0.4 × 0.7 mm, matrix = 384x384 pixels, 12 slices.

optic nerve sheath, and retro-orbital fat across 11 participants are also presented in **Table 1**. Although the coefficient of variation across participants were substantial, at an individual level, the CNRs between adjacent tissues were sufficient to distinguish them in all participants (see **Fig. 7**C). The mean CNRs between vitreous and lens, vitreous and choroid, optic nerve and subarachnoid space, subarachnoid space and nerve sheath, and nerve sheath and orbital fat are presented in **Table 2**. In one participant, susceptibility artifact prevented the lens from being resolved.

Experiment 5

Coronal T2 imaging is optional for quantitative imaging of retrobulbar ocular anatomy

A significant advantage of MRI is the ability to visualize structures behind the eyeball *in vivo*. We exploited this and conducted T2-weighted measurements of the retrobulbar ocular anatomy (**Fig. 8**). After the optic nerve exits the eyeball, it becomes myelinated and effectively doubles in diameter at about 2 to 3 mm behind the eye. As it travels posteriorly to the optic chiasm, the optic nerve is surrounded by an subarachnoid space (filled with fluid, contiguous with cerebrospinal fluid), which is surrounded by the optic nerve sheath (membrane). The clinical application here is the ability to simultaneously measure these three compartments, which can become differentially compromised in disease (eg, smaller optic nerve diameter in glaucoma,[4] increased fluid-filled subarachnoid space and/or optic nerve sheath diameter with raised intracranial pressure[5]). However, these three structures have not always been able to be distinguished from one another and the retro-orbital fat using conventional

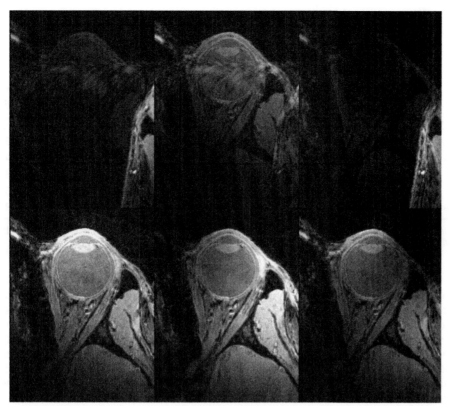

Fig. 11. Uncombined images of the six individual receive coils obtained with a 3D GRE from a left eye of a healthy 26-year-old man. Supporting the action to only acquire data from the three coils positioned closely to the eye of interest. Six-channel TX/RX eye coil array (297 MHz, icoil, MRI.TOOLS GmbH, Berlin, Germany).

magnetic field strengths and head or orbital RF coils.[6] Although some data from 3 T MRI have shown promise in distinguishing between optic nerve, subarachnoid space, and optic nerve sheath,[7,8] it is hampered by the need for either low-resolution images or thick slices (>2 mm[8]) to achieve enough contrast and signal to visualize the optic nerve. For experiment five seen in

Table 1
SNR Values for the Different Ocular Tissues

Anatomical Region	Coronal T2-Weighted TSE			Axial T2-Weighted TSE			Axial T1 GRE with Fat Saturation		
	SNR	Std	COV (%)	SNR	Std	COV (%)	SNR	Std	COV (%)
Artifact	7	2	24	12	5	41	7	1	20
Lens	—	—	—	16	5	32	182	72	39
vit	—	—	—	229	42	18	110	46	42
chor	—	—	—	37	13	35	153	54	35
Optic nerve	18	8	45	28	10	35	98	46	47
ss	37	10	26	67	18	27	119	49	41
ons	18	7	38	31	14	46	87	43	49
Fat	79	23	29	131	33	26	56	22	39

Abbreviations: chor, choroid; COV, coefficient of variation; on, optic nerve; ons, optic nerve sheath; ss, subarachnoid space; vit, vitreous humour.

Table 2
CNR Values for the Different Ocular Tissues

Anatomical Region	Coronal T2-Weighted TSE			Axial T2-Weighted TSE			Axial T1 GRE with Fat Saturation		
	CNR	Std	COV (%)	CNR	Std	COV (%)	CNR	Std	COV (%)
vit to lens	—	—	—	213	41	19	72	70	97
vit to chor	—	—	—	192	36	19	44	20	46
on to ss	20	11	58	39	16	42	20	17	85
ss to ons	19	9	46	36	13	38	32	20	64
ons to fat	60	23	38	100	27	27	31	27	85

Abbreviations: chor, choroid; COV, coefficient of variation; on, optic nerve; ons, optic nerve sheath; ss, subarachnoid space; vit, vitreous humour.

Fig. 8, the use of sub-millimeter (0.7 mm) partial volume artifact is minimized to enable more accurate demarcation of the retrobulbar optic nerve and its surrounding anatomy.[23] The SNRs (see **Table 1**) of the optic nerve, subarachnoid space, and nerve sheath were 18 (45%), 37 (26%), and 18 (38%), respectively. However, the CNRs (see **Table 2**) between the subarachnoid space, and nerve and sheath were 20 (58%) and 19 (46%), respectively. The CNRs in all subjects were above the Rose criteria[24] of 5 for adequate detection of boundaries.

Experiment 6

Axial T2 imaging is optimal for differentiating positions of gaze that create tension on the optic nerve

The ability of MRI to view the trajectory of the optic nerve behind the eye has allowed technology in conjunction with measures of strain and tension to quantify mechanical forces on the optic nerve.[8,9] Typically, the eye can achieve a wide range of duction (rotation of the eye on the vertical or horizontal axis) of up to 60°.[10] It is thought that the outer connective tissue coat of the optic nerve, the optic nerve sheath, can exert significant mechanical force on the optic nerve head and peripapillary vascular tissue when the eye undergoes duction. Repetitive eye movements and therefore repetitive strain on the optic nerve as it enters the eye have therefore been proposed as a mechanism of damage to susceptible optic nerves in diseases such as glaucoma.[8] In **Fig. 9A–C**, showing experiment 6 results, the high-resolution axial T2 images of the eye and its optic nerve during horizontal duction (right and left gaze) relative to a neutral position can

be easily visualized. These high-resolution images have adequate signal and contrast (Rose[24] criteria >5) to easily quantify the gaze angle, optic nerve length, anterior-posterior depth, and ocular axial length. In addition, with fat saturation (see **Fig. 9D**), the cerebrospinal fluid surrounding the optic nerve can be clearly identified and quantified (if required). The variation in echo time appears to have no obvious visual effect on tissue differentiation as seen in **Fig. 10**. The decision to adopt the echo time of 45 ms was seen as a compromise of an appropriate echo time for T2 image weighting, without the signal loss that is known to arise from increasing the echo time, because of T2* dephasing.[13,25]

Highest resolution and contrast anatomic imaging of the eye and orbit can be achieved with clinically available pulse sequence technology

As clinical translation at 7T becomes more prominent, a reoccurring question is, can the application of sequences developed by research sites be implemented successfully clinically? In this study, all sequences used are product sequences, so they can be adapted to a clinical setting; however, consideration of coil choice would be significant. In order to benefit from the improved SNR and CNR that are attainable at high field, a dedicated eye coil would potentially be required. As discussed, the susceptibility artifact when scanning this region of the head must to be treated with caution and care. The susceptibility artifact and sequence time are just two of the factors that may hinder the move to advanced imaging techniques such as diffusion, fMRI, arterial spin labeling, or susceptibility imaging without input and adoption of current research sequences.[26]

SUMMARY

In conclusion, we have shown that the synergistic combination of a dedicated phased array eye RF coil, a field strength of 7T, parallel image reconstruction, and careful participant preparation allows for high-resolution and contrast MRI images of the entire eye and orbit to be acquired. We believe these to be some of the highest resolution *in vivo* human MRI eye images published to date with protocols readily available on clinical 7T MRI scanners. We were able to image the retrobulbar optic nerve in 2D and 3D while avoiding significant motion artifact by adopting appropriate visual fixation and eye preparation techniques, the feasibility of which was demonstrated by reproducing high-quality images across a cohort of healthy emmetropic participants.

ACKNOWLEDGMENTS

The authors thank MRI.TOOLS GmbH, Berlin, Germany, for guidance in implementing coil characteristics during pilot testing and Mr Trevor McQuilland and Mr Edward Green at the Department of Biomedical Engineering, University of Melbourne, for the design and fabrication of the coil stabiliser. The authors acknowledge the facilities and the scientific and technical assistance of the Australian National Imaging Facility at the Melbourne Brain Centre Imaging Unit. This work was supported by a research collaboration agreement with Siemens Healthineers.

DISCLOSURE

A.M. McKendrick receives research support from Heidelberg Engineering GmBH. Funding was provided by Melbourne Neuroscience Institute Fellowship (B.N. Nguyen); The University of Melbourne McKenzie Fellowship (J.O. Cleary); and Melbourne Neuroscience Institute Interdisciplinary Seed Funding Grant (A.M. McKendrick, B.V. Bui, and R.J. Ordidge). The National Imaging Facility supports the 7T system at the Melbourne Brain Center Imaging Unit and the MRI Facility Fellow (B.A. Moffat).

SUPPLEMENTARY DATA

Supplementary data related to this article can be found online at https://doi.org/10.1016/j.mric.2020.09.004.

REFERENCES

1. Jonas J, Xu L. Histological changes of high axial myopia. Eye (Lond) 2013;28:113–7.

2. Kuo AN, Verkicharla PK, McNabb RP, et al. Posterior Eye Shape Measurement With Retinal OCT Compared to MRI. Invest Ophthalmol Vis Sci 2016; 57(9):OCT196–203.

3. Smith G, Atchison DA, Iskander DR, et al. Mathematical models for describing the shape of the in vitro unstretched human crystalline lens. Vision Res 2009;49(20):2442–52.

4. Moffat BA, Landman KA, Truscott RJ, et al. Age-related changes in the kinetics of water transport in normal human lenses. Exp Eye Res 1999;69(6): 663–9.

5. Moffat BA, Atchison DA, Pope JM. Explanation of the lens paradox. Optom Vis Sci 2002;79(3):148–50.

6. Christoforidis JB, Wassenaar PA, Christoforidis GA, et al. Retrobulbar vasculature using 7-T magnetic resonance imaging with dedicated eye surface coil. Graefes Arch Clin Exp Ophthalmol 2013; 251(1):271–7.

7. Jones CE, Atchison DA, Pope JM. Changes in lens dimensions and refractive index with age and accommodation. Optom Vis Sci 2007;84(10):990–5.

8. Niendorf T, Paul K, Graessl A, et al. [Ophthalmological imaging with ultrahigh field magnetic resonance tomography: technical innovations and frontier applications]. Klin Monbl Augenheilkd 2014;231(12): 1187–95.

9. Liebo GB, Fuller ML, Witte R, et al. High-Resolution Volumetric MR Ocular Imaging at 3T: A Pictorial Review With Ophthalmic and Sonographic Correlation. Neurographics 2016;6:281–91.

10. Khurana A, Eisenhut CA, Wan W, et al. Comparison of the diagnostic value of MR imaging and ophthalmoscopy for the staging of retinoblastoma. Eur Radiol 2013;23(5):1271–80.

11. Harrigan RL, Smith AK, Mawn LA, et al. Short Term Reproducibility of a High Contrast 3-D Isotropic Optic Nerve Imaging Sequence in Healthy Controls. Proc SPIE Int Soc Opt Eng 2016;9783:97831L.

12. Kasthurirangan S, Markwell EL, Atchison DA, et al. In vivo study of changes in refractive index distribution in the human crystalline lens with age and accommodation. Invest Ophthalmol Vis Sci 2008; 49(6):2531–40.

13. Pohmann R, Speck O, Scheffler K. Signal-to-noise ratio and MR tissue parameters in human brain imaging at 3, 7, and 9.4 tesla using current receive coil arrays. Magn Reson Med 2016;75(2):801–9.

14. Richdale K, Wassenaar P, Teal Bluestein K, et al. 7 Tesla MR imaging of the human eye in vivo. J Magn Reson Imaging 2009;30(5):924–32.

15. Graessl A, Muhle M, Schwerter M, et al. Ophthalmic magnetic resonance imaging at 7 T using a 6-channel transceiver radiofrequency coil array in healthy subjects and patients with intraocular masses. Invest Radiol 2014;49(5):260–70.

16. Wezel J, Garpebring A, Webb AG, et al. Automated eye blink detection and correction method for clinical MR eye imaging. Magn Reson Med 2017; 78(1):165–71.

17. Zhang Y, Peng Q, Kiel JW, et al. Magnetic Resonance Imaging of Vascular Oxygenation Changes during Hyperoxia and Carbogen Challenges in the Human Retina. Invest Ophthalmol Vis Sci 2011; 52(1):286–91.

18. Singh AD, Platt SM, Lystad L, et al. Optic Nerve Assessment Using 7-Tesla Magnetic Resonance Imaging. Ocul Oncol Pathol 2016;2(3):178–80.

19. Bert RJ, Patz S, Ossiani M, et al. High-resolution MR imaging of the human eye 2005. Acad Radiol 2006; 13(3):368–78.

20. Harrigan RL, Plassard AJ, Bryan FW, et al. Disambiguating the optic nerve from the surrounding cerebrospinal fluid: Application to MS-related atrophy. Magn Reson Med 2016;75(1):414–22.

21. Mashima Y, Oshitari K, Imamura Y, et al. High-Resolution Magnetic Resonance Imaging of the Intraorbital Optic Nerve and Subarachnoid Space in Patients With Papilledema and Optic Atrophy. Arch Ophthalmol 1996;114(10):1197–203.

22. Demer JL. Optic nerve sheath as a novel mechanical load on the globe in ocular duction. Invest Ophthalmol Vis Sci 2016;57(4):1826–38.

23. Nguyen BN, Cleary JO, Glarin R, et al. Normative retrobulbar measurements of the optic nerve using ultra high field magnetic resonance imaging. Invest Ophthalmol Vis Sci 2019;60(9):6109.

24. Watts R, Wang Y. k-space interpretation of the Rose Model: noise limitation on the detectable resolution in MRI. Magn Reson Med 2002;48(3):550–4.

25. Cao Z, Park J, Cho Z-H, et al. Numerical evaluation of image homogeneity, signal-to-noise ratio, and specific absorption rate for human brain imaging at 1.5, 3, 7, 10.5, and 14T in an 8-channel transmit/receive array. J Magn Reson Imaging 2015; 41(5):1432–9.

26. Paul K, Huelnhagen T, Oberacker E, et al. Multiband diffusion-weighted MRI of the eye and orbit free of geometric distortions using a RARE-EPI hybrid. NMR Biomed 2018;31(3):e3872.

Musculoskeletal MR Imaging Applications at Ultra-High (7T) Field Strength

Rajiv G. Menon, PhD[a],*, Gregory Chang, MD[b], Ravinder R. Regatte, PhD[a]

KEYWORDS

• Ultrahigh field (UHF) MR imaging • 7 T • Musculoskeletal MR imaging • Cartilage • Bone

KEY POINTS

- Ultrahigh field (UHF) offers enhanced signal-to-noise ratio (SNR) and contrast-to-noise ratio (CNR), and provides unique morphologic and functional information in vivo, not available at lower field strengths, and presents several opportunities and challenges in quantitative musculoskeletal imaging.
- Several musculoskeletal applications at UHF, including morphologic applications, T_1, T_2, and $T_{1\rho}$ mapping, multinuclear applications with sodium, phosphorus, and spectroscopy provide unique advantages at UHF.
- UHF also represents several technical challenges and is not suited for all imaging applications.
- Developing robust new techniques and applications tailored for UHF is critical for widespread clinical adoption.

INTRODUCTION

The approval of ultrahigh field (7T) magnetic resonance scanners for clinical use by the US Food and Drug Administration, and the European regulatory authority have opened the doors for more widespread clinical adoption[1,2] particularly with the release of clinical UHF scanners by MR vendors. Although most of the clinical MR systems are 1.5, and 3T systems, several large hospitals and academic research centers have explored musculoskeletal MR applications at UHF.[3–9] UHF 7T scanners provide a unique set of advantages over lower field strength scanners, but they also come with a set of technical and safety challenges. The choice of whether to use a UHF scanner is more nuanced and based on the intended application, and thus, it is important to understand the advantages, disadvantages, and current challenges of 7T systems for clinical use.

Advantages and Disadvantages

Increase of the main field strength, B_0, to 7T has several advantages:

- With the increasing B_0 field strength, increased numbers of protons are polarized, resulting in a net increase in the magnetization M_0.
- The signal-to-noise ratio (SNR) scales with the square of B_0 hence more than doubles at 7T.[10] This gain in SNR can be used in multiple ways such as acquiring images with increased spatial resolution, increased temporal resolution, or scan time reductions.
- Contrast-to-noise ratio (CNR), which is in many cases a more relevant parameter for diagnostic purposes in terms of detection of lesions. Applications such as functional MR imaging and quantitative susceptibility mapping gain with enhanced CNR due to susceptibility increases at UHF fields.

[a] Department of Radiology, New York University Langone Health, Bernard and Irene Schwartz Center for Biomedical Imaging, 660 First Avenue 4th Floor, New York, NY 10016, USA; [b] Department of Radiology, New York University Langone Health, Bernard and Irene Schwartz Center for Biomedical Imaging, 660 First Avenue, Room 334, New York, NY 10016, USA
* Corresponding author.
E-mail address: Rajiv.menon@nyulangone.org

Magn Reson Imaging Clin N Am 29 (2021) 117–127
https://doi.org/10.1016/j.mric.2020.09.008

- Spectral resolution is enhanced at 7T and allows better identification of metabolites.[11]
- In addition, multinuclear applications including ^{23}Na, ^{31}P, ^{17}O, and ^{13}C stand to gain at UHF.

The increased B_0 strength also presents unique technical challenges. The B_1 field required scales quadratically with B_0 field strength. Although this requires increased B_1 power to achieve similar flip angles compared with lower field strengths, this affects a key safety measure of tissue heating called specific absorption rate (SAR).[12] The radiofrequency (RF) wavelength in tissues reduces from ~35 cm to ~15 cm from 3T to 7T, resulting in decreased ability of RF pulses to penetrate tissue and thus causes flip angle variability across the sample. In addition, the use of body coils for transmitting RF pulses becomes impractical at 7T. One option is to use RF transmit phase arrays, but this causes interference and cross-talk of RF waves resulting in "hot spots." This makes imaging large organs challenging. Currently 7T applications focus on the use of birdcage coils that enclose the region of interest and are primarily used for neuroimaging and imaging extremities. Another drawback is that at 7T, there are significant variations in receiving B_1 inhomogeneity and require accurate flip angle maps and receive sensitivity maps. Finally, at higher fields, relaxation values of tissue changes. Generally, T_1 values increase,[13] and T_2[14] and T_2^* values decrease due to increased susceptibility.

Although the use of UHF has distinct advantages and many drawbacks, the use of UHF should be determined by the intended application. **Table 1** summarizes the pros and cons of using UHF for musculoskeletal imaging applications. Some applications have definite advantages and provide more information than lower powered scanners, hence are definitely recommended. Other applications where technical challenges tip the scales may not be beneficial to use UHF currently. As these technical challenges are solved, more applications may become feasible to use at UHF. This review focuses on the emergence of UHF for musculoskeletal MR imaging and surveys recent advances in MR imaging techniques for musculoskeletal applications.

MR IMAGING TECHNIQUES FOR MINIMUM SHIFT KEYING APPLICATIONS AT 7T
Application 1: Morphologic Imaging

With SNR and CNR enhancements at UHF, morphologic imaging provides greater details of biological structure. UHF allows ultrahigh-resolution imaging of cartilage with better structural visualization. The improved contrast at 7T allows better segmentation of the cartilage structures. Furthermore, the reduction in voxel size minimizes partial volume artifacts. This allows for improved measurements of thickness and volume in cartilage structures. The sequences typically used for morphologic imaging are conventional spin echo (SE) and gradient echo (GRE) sequences and 3D-SE and -GRE sequences, with fat suppression.[15] GRE-based sequences such as spoiled gradient recalled echo or fast low-angle shot (FLASH) produce hyperintense cartilage signal and good contrast between surrounding structures for segmentation algorithms.[16] High-resolution knee cartilage imaging at $254 \times 254 \times 1000 \ \mu m^3$ was demonstrated using a 3D-FLASH sequence by Regatte and Schweitzer.[9] Chang and colleagues showed clinical feasibility studies in the hip using custom-built coils and UHF at a resolution of $230 \times 230 \times 1500 \ \mu m^3$.[17] More recently, Chebrolu and colleagues have demonstrated correction algorithms for coil-induced nonuniformity using uniform combined reconstruction (UNICORN) algorithm (**Fig. 1**).[18]

Increased SNR in UHF allows the enhanced visualization and quantitative assessment of bone structures in the tibia, knee, hip, and wrist. The size of individual trabeculae is about 100 to 150 μm, with relatively large distances between trabeculae on the order of 300 to 800 μm.[10] Susceptibility differences between the trabecular bone and bone marrow result in broadening of the trabecular signal, especially in GRE sequences. These susceptibility effects proportionally increase with field strength, with UHF providing enhanced visualization of the small trabeculae, which would have otherwise disappeared from partial volume effects.[19,20] Examples of trabecular bone imaging of the tibia,[9,21] knee,[22,23] hip,[17] and wrist[24,25] at 7T demonstrate the feasibility of imaging bone to assess microarchitecture. **Fig. 2** shows the application of imaging bone microarchitecture in the hip in osteoporotic patients. With in-plane resolutions of 100 to 200 μm^2 available, assessments such as percent bone volume, trabecular thickness, trabecular spacing, and trabecular number have shown good correlation with μCT.[17]

Application 2: T_2 and T_2^* Mapping

Quantitative T_2 mapping is useful to understand changes in collagen, as it reflects the interaction of water in the extracellular matrix. In cartilage, T_2 maps reflects the integrity of the collagen matrix, glycosaminoglycan (GAG) content, and

Table 1
Pros and cons for musculoskeletal MR imaging at ultrahigh field

Characteristic	Trend (at UHF)	Advantage	Disadvantage
SNR	Increases	Higher resolution imaging, more detailed information	None
CNR	Increases	Increased lesion detection, diagnostic value	None
SAR	Increases	None	Limits imaging sequence capability, longer scan times
Physiologic effects	Increases	None	Dizziness, nausea, metallic taste
Relaxation times (T_1, T_2, T_3)	T_1 increases, T_2 decreases, T_2* decreases		Longer scan time
RF field uniformity	Reduces	None	Flip angle variation, poor inversion
Susceptibility effects	Increases	Beneficial for BOLD, T_2* imaging	Geometric distortions, intravoxel dephasing
Chemical shift	Increases	Beneficial for CEST, MRS applications	Fat/water, metabolite misregistration

An overview of the advantages and disadvantages of imaging at UHF for musculoskeletal imaging applications.
    From Ladd ME, Bachert P, Meyerspeer M, et al. Pros and cons of ultra-high-field MRI/MRS for human application. Progress in Nuclear Magnetic Resonance Spectroscopy. 2018 Dec; 109(1):1-50; with permission.

hydration.[26] The earliest events in osteoarthritis (OA) include the degradation of the collagen matrix and loss of GAG.[27] Several clinical studies have used T_2 mapping as outcome measures to assess OA risk.[28,29] At 7T, consistent with lower T_2 values at UHF, T_2 maps exhibited lower values and lower stratification across the cartilage, which is useful in the assessment of cartilage.[30] For T_2 mapping, multiecho spin echo (MESE)[30,31] sequences are used. A study by Chang and colleagues looking at surgically repaired knee cartilage with healthy controls, and a study by Domayer and colleagues comparing postsurgical ankle cartilage with controls was able to distinguish cartilage repair tissue from healthy cartilage at UHF, demonstrating its ability to detect altered collagen composition.[32,33] In 2014, the 3D-triple echo steady state technique was reported as an alternative to the MESE sequence, a technique for efficient T_2 mapping with low SAR, good spatial coverage, and insensitivity to B_0 and B_1 inhomogeneities.[34,35] Two studies, one by Juras and colleagues and another by Kraff and colleagues, have demonstrated its utility for T_2 mapping.[36,37] **Fig. 2**A–F shows the comparison of T2 mapping at 3T and 7T in a patient with a traumatic cartilage lesion at baseline and at a 12-month follow-up scan.[38]

The T_2 decay times of structures such as tendons, ligaments, bone, and menisci are very short

(8 μs–500 μs) and are virtually invisible or low signal intensity in clinical sequences. After it was originally proposed,[39] techniques were developed to allow T_2* mapping using ultrashort echo time (UTE) imaging. Using a combination of radial readouts, ramp sampling, short duration RF pulses, and unique sampling strategies several new techniques were developed to visualize short T_2 structures.[40–42] At 7T, the SNR for UTE-based sequences gets a boost, and tissues are visualized better. On the other hand, a challenge is that these short T_2 decays become even shorter at UHF. This has to be accounted for when designing imaging sequences for UHF. Krug and colleagues demonstrated UTE imaging of the bone at 7T.[43] Juras and colleagues showed that Achilles tendon can be imaged in controls and patients at UHF.[44] More recently, Larson and colleagues demonstrated knee and ankle imaging at 7T performed using UTE and zero echo time (ZTE).[45] Welsch and colleagues demonstrated the comparison of T_2 and T_2* maps at 3T and 7T.[30] **Fig. 2**G and H shows the comparison of T_2*-weighted images of the Achilles tendon at 3T and 7T, respectively.[44]

Application 3: $T_{1\rho}$ Mapping

$T_{1\rho}$ is sensitive to low-frequency interactions related to chemical exchange between extracellular water and other macromolecules.[46,47] At HF,

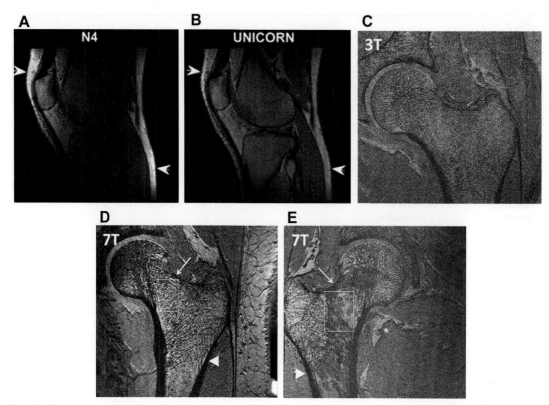

Fig. 1. Morphologic imaging. Figure 1A shows reconstruction without correction at 7T and (*B*) shows the improvement in reconstruction at 7T, when MR image intensity inhomogeneities are accounted for using the UNI-CORN algorithm. Figure (*C*) shows hip bone microarchitecture in an osteoporotic patient at 3T, where the trabeculae are not clearly seen. At 7T, clear assessments of the trabeculae in an osteopenia patient can be done as shown in (*D*). (*E*) shows fewer visible trabeculae proximal femoral diaphysis in an osteoporotic patient (*box*) and thinning of mineralized bone (*arrows*). (*From* Chang G, Deniz CM, Honig S, et al. MRI of the hip at 7T: feasibility of bone microarchitecture, high-resolution cartilage, and clinical imaging. J Magn Reson Imaging 2014; 39(6): 1384-93; with permission. And *From* Chebrolu VV, Kollasch PD, Deshpande V, et al. Uniform combined reconstruction of multichannel 7T knee MRI receive coil data without the use of a reference scan. J Magn Reson Imaging 2019; 50(5): 1534-44; with permission.)

$T_{1\rho}$ mapping has been extensively used to quantify proteoglycan content in articular cartilage.[48–50] At UHF, B_1 and B_0 inhomogeneities and long spin-lock RF pulses and SAR limitations make it challenging to implement $T_{1\rho}$ imaging pulse sequences. Singh and colleagues demonstrated the feasibility of $T_{1\rho}$ mapping at UHF in healthy controls and patients.[51] They were able to distinguish between healthy and pathologic cartilage $T_{1\rho}$ values. They noted that $T_{1\rho}$ values at 7T were significantly lower compared with 3T. **Fig. 3** shows the $T_{1\rho}$ results obtained in the study. Another study by Wyatt and colleagues compared $T_{1\rho}$ at 3T and 7T with a group of patients with OA and controls. They demonstrated increased $T_{1\rho}$ values in the patients with OA and significant differences between controls and patients with OA at 7T. The results they reported is shown in **Fig. 3**.[52]

Application 4: Chemical Exchange Saturation Transfer

Chemical exchange occurs between bulk water and protons bound to macromolecules. Chemical exchange saturation transfer (CEST) allows the indirect measurement of these exchangeable macromolecular protons by saturating the bound macromolecular protons using a series of off-resonance RF pulses and then observe the reduction of water signal intensity. This reduction in signal intensity is proportional to the local macromolecular content. For cartilage, GAG CEST (gagCEST) is a technique that allows the quantification of the GAG content in the macromolecular pool by applying off-resonance irradiation to the protons in the hydroxyl groups of cartilage GAG, which was first demonstrated in vivo at 3T[53] and

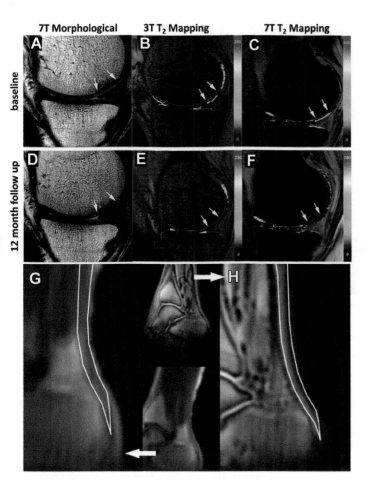

baseline

12 month follow up

Fig. 2. T2 mapping and T2* imaging. Figure 2A–F shows an example of a patient with a traumatic cartilage lesion, where the hyperintense region became hypointense over time. (A–C) shows morphologic, T2 mapping at 3T, and T2 mapping at 7T at baseline, and (D–F) shows the corresponding images in the same patient at a 12-month follow-up scan. (G–H) shows T2* weighted images of the Achilles tendon using a UTE sequence at 3T [(G)] and 7T [(H)]. SNR and CNR are significantly higher at 7T. (*From* Juras V, Schreiner M, Laurent D, et al. The comparison of the performance of 3T and 7T T2 mapping for untreated low-grade cartilage lesions. Magn Reson Imaging 2019; 55: 86-92; with permission. And *From* Juras V, Zbyn S, Pressl C, et al. Regional variations of T(2)* in healthy and pathologic achilles tendon in vivo at 7 Tesla: preliminary results. Magn Reson Med 2012; 68(5): 1607-13; with permission.)

was later demonstrated in vivo at 7T.[54] The hydroxyl protons resonate at a frequency very close to bulk water at 0 to 1.5 ppm. Hence gagCEST becomes unsuitable at field strengths of 3T or below where frequency separation is too small, and causes RF spillover, thus impairing its quantification at or below 3T. At higher fields, the RF spillover is considerably reduced, making it a viable technique at 7T. **Fig. 4** shows that at 3T there is a negligible observable gagCEST signal, but consistent gagCEST observable signal of more than 5% is obtained at 7T.[55] Several recent

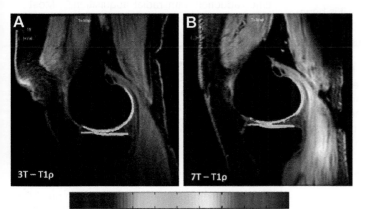

3T – T1ρ   7T – T1ρ

0   8   16   24   32   40   48   56   64   72   80

Fig. 3. T$_{1\rho}$ mapping of knee cartilage. Figure (A) shows T$_{1\rho}$ mapping of the knee cartilage at 3T and 7T (B) in a healthy subject. (*From* Wyatt C, Guha A, Venkatachari A, et al. Improved differentiation between knees with cartilage lesions and controls using 7T relaxation time mapping. J Orthop Translat 2015; 3(4): 197-204; with permission.)

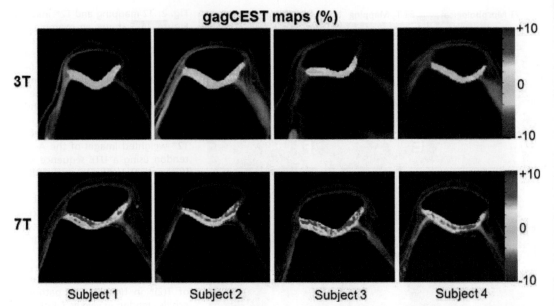

Fig. 4. gagCEST comparison in knee cartilage. Corrected knee gagCEST maps from 4 healthy volunteers at 3 T (top row) and 7 T (bottom row), respectively. (*From* Singh A, Haris M, Cai K, et al. Chemical exchange saturation transfer magnetic resonance imaging of human knee cartilage at 3 T and 7 T. Magn Reson Med 2012; 68(2): 588-94; with permission.)

studies have demonstrated the feasibility of using gagCEST at 7T in controls and patients.[56–59] **Fig. 4** shows the comparison of gagCEST in the knee cartilage at 3T and 7T, following B_0 inhomogeneity correction[55] (see **Fig. 4**).

Application 5: Sodium Imaging

Sodium is widely present in all tissue types and is a desirable imaging target to glean critical metabolic information. In cartilage, Na^+ cation balance the negatively charged GAG and is an early indicator of the health of the cartilage.[60] There are numerous advantages of using ^{23}Na as a tool to assess biochemical composition at UHF:

- SNR scales with B_0 for ^{23}Na, hence it is beneficial at 7T.
- The wavelength for ^{23}Na is much higher compared with protons, hence imaging at UHF is easier, as there are fewer B_1 inhomogeneity and B_0 susceptibility issues.
- The T_1 of ^{23}Na is governed by quadrupolar interactions, hence T_1 values do not increase with B_0 strength. This allows for more signal averages to be obtained within the same amount of time.
- ^{23}Na has high specificity and does not require contrast agent.

Imaging using ^{23}Na is not without challenges, as it requires higher field strength to work feasibly.

Lower MR sensitivity to ^{23}Na compared with ^1H and lower in vivo concentrations compared with protons result in a net effect that the ^{23}Na signal is 4000 times lower than that of protons. In addition, multinuclear capability in the scanners with custom RF coil development requirements are current barriers to entry for more wide-spread use of ^{23}Na imaging.[61,62] To improve SNR, center-out non-Cartesian trajectories such as fermat looped, orthogonally encoded trajectory,[63] variable density spirals, and radial trajectories,[64] 3D cones[65] have been implemented. ^{23}Na has a short T_2 relaxation time, hence UTE sequences are most suited, such as sweep imaging with Fourier transform,[66] ZTE,[67] and point-wise encoding time reduction with radial acquisition.[42] Most of the sequences here use non-Cartesian trajectories and subsequently use a regridding technique with iterative compressed sensing reconstruction methods.[68] Concentration of ^{23}Na in healthy cartilage is 250 to 350 mM and in osteoarthritic cartilage starts to go less than 250 mM.[69] At 7T, a few studies have shown the use of ^{23}Na in quantifying GAG content in OA and cartilage repair[70,71] (**Fig. 5**).

Sodium Metabolic Imaging of Skeletal Muscle

^{23}Na imaging has significant potential in providing insight into muscular physiology and disorders, but more work needs to be done at UHF. In

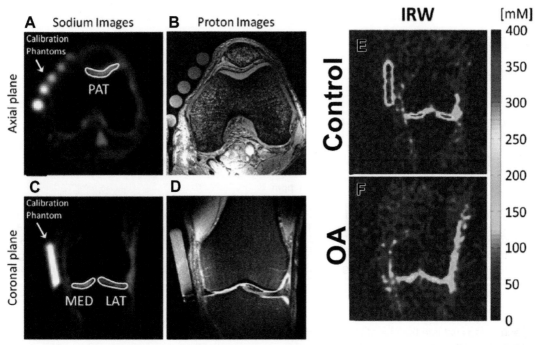

Fig. 5. Sodium imaging. Figures (*A*) and (*B*) show representative sodium and proton images patellar cartilage. Figure (*C*) and (*D*) show representative sodium and proton images of femorotibial medial and femorotibial lateral cartilage. Figure (*E*) shows sodium concentration maps from one control subject and (*F*) one patient with knee osteoarthritis (*OA*). Note the higher difference in sodium concentration between femorotibial medial and femorotibial lateral regions of control subject and patient with knee osteoarthritis. (*From* Madelin G, Babb J, Xia D, et al. Articular cartilage: evaluation with fluid-suppressed 7.0-T sodium MR imaging in subjects with and subjects without osteoarthritis. Radiology 2013; 268(2): 481-91; with permission.)

skeletal muscles, ^{23}Na is mostly concentrated in the extracellular region. When an action potential is generated, the Na$^+$/K$^+$ ATPase mechanism causes the rapid influx of ^{23}Na into the cells, leading to muscular contraction. Altered Na$^+$/K$^+$ ATPase activity has been implicated in several metabolic pathologies.[72] The applications of ^{23}Na imaging have shown their feasibility in several studies including diabetes,[73] muscular channelopathy,[74] and hypertension.[75]

Application 6: Phosphorus Spectroscopy and ^{31}P-MR Imaging

^{31}Phosphorus MR spectroscopy (^{31}P-MRS) has been used since a long time as a technique to assess bioenergetics in skeletal muscle at lower fields.[76,77] It can detect phosphocreatine (PCr), inorganic phosphates (Pi), and other phosphate groups. ^{31}P-MRS gives a tool for investigating muscle metabolism in resting and postexercise states and determination of cellular pH. ^{31}P-MRS and ^{31}P-MR imaging have been used in several applications including mitochondrial diseases,[78] metabolic disorders,[79] diabetes,[80] peripheral artery disease,[81] and muscle injury.[82]

At UHF, there are some unique advantages for imaging and spectroscopy of ^{31}P. Along with the increase in SNR, and spectral resolution, the ^{31}P T$_1$ relaxation time reduces, which speeds up acquisition time. Bogner and colleagues demonstrated in their study that at 7T, the ^{31}P-SNR is twice that of 3T.[83] Prodromos and colleagues developed, at 3T and 7T, a spectrally selective ^{31}P-MRS technique that allowed simultaneous localized measurement of *phosphocreatine* (PCr) resynthesis rates at rest and following exercise[84,85] (**Fig. 6**). Hooijmans and colleagues showed using ^{31}P-MRS that phosphodiester levels are elevated in patients with Duchenne muscular dystrophy.[86] Korzowski and Bachert developed a ^{31}P echo-planar spectroscopic imaging method at UHF.[87] Schmid and colleagues developed a method for the simultaneous measurement of PCr and pH in calf muscles following exercise.[88]

DISCUSSION AND SUMMARY

At present it is unclear whether improved image quality (higher SNR, CNR, resolution) at UHF increases diagnostic accuracy. More clinical studies

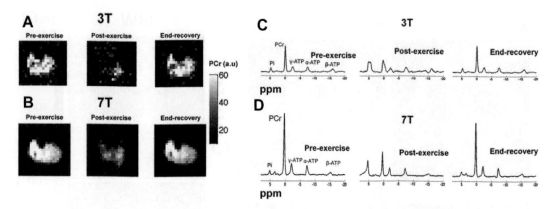

Fig. 6. ^{31}P-MRS and MR imaging. (*A*) and (*B*) show ^{31}P imaging pre- and postexercise cross-sectional slice of the lower leg muscles of the same subject before the beginning and at the end of the exercise, as well as at the end of the recovery period at 3T and at 7T. MR spectra of the same volunteer pre- and postexercise. Almost 3-fold increase in the SNR from 3T (*C*) to 7T (*D*) is observed, after normalization. (*From* Parasoglou P, Xia D, Chang G, et al. Dynamic three-dimensional imaging of phosphocreatine recovery kinetics in the human lower leg muscles at 3T and 7T: a preliminary study. NMR Biomed 2013; 26(3): 348-56; with permission.)

are required to evaluate the use of UHF as a diagnostic differentiator compared with lower field systems. Mitigating safety concerns of UHF, custom pulse sequence optimizations, development of new RF coils and hardware for imaging, and overcoming the challenges with UHF imaging are some of the requirements that need to be met for more widespread acceptance of UHF as a diagnostic clinical imaging tool.

At UHF, the behavior of tissues, as well as B_1 and B_0 change. These changes produce several challenges but also present several opportunities in musculoskeletal imaging that may be developed to create a toolset of clinical diagnostic tools not available until now. There are several potential diagnostic applications at 7T that are not feasible at lower fields or perform better at UHF such as sodium imaging, gagCEST, T_2 mapping, clinical ^{31}P spectroscopy, and imaging. There is opportunity to develop a useful diagnostic toolset based on the unique changes that UHF brings. Developing useful and robust new methods unique to UHF are critical for the development of the 7T clinical human systems as a diagnostic tool for quantitative musculoskeletal applications.

CLINICS CARE POINTS

- For musculoskeletal imaging, 7T offers opportunities for increased information from higher SNR, CNR, increased spectral resolution and multi-nuclear imaging.
- Disadvantages of higher field in the form of increased SAR, relaxation time changes, B1 and B0 inhomogeneities and their impact

must be considered for particular applications.
- The challenges represent future opportunity to improve techniques for impactful clinical workflows.

ACKNOWLEDGMENTS

This study was supported by NIH grants R21-AR075259-01A1, R01 AR076328, R01 AR067156, and R01 AR068966, and was performed under the rubric of the Center of Advanced Imaging Innovation and Research (CAI2R), a NIBIB Biomedical Technology Resource Center (NIH P41 EB017183).

DISCLOSURE

The authors have nothing to disclose.

REFERENCES

1. Press Release. FDA clears first 7T magnetic resonance imaging device. Available at: https://www.fda.gov/NewsEvents/Newsroom/PressAnnouncements/ucm580154.htm. Accessed February 1, 2018.
2. Press Release: With 7 Tesla scanner Magnetom Terra, Siemens Healthineers introduces new clinical field strength in MR imaging. Available at: https://www.siemens.com/press/PR2017080391HCEN. Accessed February 1, 2018.
3. Alizai H, Chang G, Regatte RR. MRI of the Musculoskeletal System: Advanced Applications using High and Ultrahigh Field MRI. Semin Musculoskelet Radiol 2015;19(4):363–74.

4. Bangerter NK, Taylor MD, Tarbox GJ, et al. Quantitative techniques for musculoskeletal MRI at 7 Tesla. Quant Imaging Med Surg 2016;6(6):715–30.

5. Dula AN, Virostko J, Shellock FG. Assessment of MRI issues at 7 T for 28 implants and other objects. AJR Am J Roentgenol 2014;202(2):401–5.

6. Karamat MI, Darvish-Molla S, Santos-Diaz A. Opportunities and Challenges of 7 Tesla Magnetic Resonance Imaging: A Review. Crit Rev Biomed Eng 2016;44(1–2):73–89.

7. Kraff O, Quick HH. 7T: Physics, safety, and potential clinical applications. J Magn Reson Imaging 2017; 46(6):1573–89.

8. Moser E, Stahlberg F, Ladd ME, et al. 7-T MR–from research to clinical applications? NMR Biomed 2012;25(5):695–716.

9. Regatte RR, Schweitzer ME. Ultra-high-field MRI of the musculoskeletal system at 7.0T. J Magn Reson Imaging 2007;25(2):262–9.

10. Krug R, Stehling C, Kelley DA, et al. Imaging of the musculoskeletal system in vivo using ultra-high field magnetic resonance at 7 T. Invest Radiol 2009;44(9):613–8.

11. Scheenen TW, Heerschap A, Klomp DW. Towards 1H-MRSI of the human brain at 7T with slice-selective adiabatic refocusing pulses. MAGMA 2008;21(1–2):95–101.

12. Collins CM, Wang Z. Calculation of radiofrequency electromagnetic fields and their effects in MRI of human subjects. Magn Reson Med 2011;65(5): 1470–82.

13. Jordan CD, Saranathan M, Bangerter NK, et al. Musculoskeletal MRI at 3.0 T and 7.0 T: a comparison of relaxation times and image contrast. Eur J Radiol 2013;82(5):734–9.

14. Pruessmann KP. Parallel imaging at high field strength: synergies and joint potential. Top Magn Reson Imaging 2004;15(4):237–44.

15. Crema MD, Roemer FW, Marra MD, et al. Articular cartilage in the knee: current MR imaging techniques and applications in clinical practice and research. Radiographics 2011;31(1):37–61.

16. Duc SR, Pfirrmann CW, Schmid MR, et al. Articular cartilage defects detected with 3D water-excitation true FISP: prospective comparison with sequences commonly used for knee imaging. Radiology 2007; 245(1):216–23.

17. Chang G, Deniz CM, Honig S, et al. MRI of the hip at 7T: feasibility of bone microarchitecture, high-resolution cartilage, and clinical imaging. J Magn Reson Imaging 2014;39(6):1384–93.

18. Chebrolu VV, Kollasch PD, Deshpande V, et al. Uniform combined reconstruction of multichannel 7T knee MRI receive coil data without the use of a reference scan. J Magn Reson Imaging 2019;50(5): 1534–44.

19. Majumdar S. Quantitative study of the susceptibility difference between trabecular bone and bone marrow: computer simulations. Magn Reson Med 1991;22(1):101–10.

20. Majumdar S, Thomasson D, Shimakawa A, et al. Quantitation of the susceptibility difference between trabecular bone and bone marrow: experimental studies. Magn Reson Med 1991;22(1):111–27.

21. Krug R, Carballido-Gamio J, Banerjee S, et al. In vivo ultra-high-field magnetic resonance imaging of trabecular bone microarchitecture at 7 T. J Magn Reson Imaging 2008;27(4):854–9.

22. Chang G, Regatte RR, Schweitzer ME. Olympic fencers: adaptations in cortical and trabecular bone determined by quantitative computed tomography. Osteoporos Int 2009;20(5):779–85.

23. Kraff O, Theysohn JM, Maderwald S, et al. MRI of the knee at 7.0 Tesla. Rofo 2007;179(12):1231–5.

24. Chang G, Friedrich KM, Wang L, et al. MRI of the wrist at 7 tesla using an eight-channel array coil combined with parallel imaging: preliminary results. J Magn Reson Imaging 2010;31(3):740–6.

25. Nobauer-Huhmann IM, Pretterklieber M, Erhart J, et al. Anatomy and variants of the triangular fibrocartilage complex and its MR appearance at 3 and 7T. Semin Musculoskelet Radiol 2012;16(2): 93–103.

26. Menezes NM, Gray ML, Hartke JR, et al. T2 and T1rho MRI in articular cartilage systems. Magn Reson Med 2004;51(3):503–9.

27. Poole AR. An introduction to the pathophysiology of osteoarthritis. Front Biosci 1999;4:D662–70.

28. Joseph GB, Baum T, Alizai H, et al. Baseline mean and heterogeneity of MR cartilage T2 are associated with morphologic degeneration of cartilage, meniscus, and bone marrow over 3 years–data from the Osteoarthritis Initiative. Osteoarthritis Cartilage 2012;20(7):727–35.

29. Lin W, Alizai H, Joseph GB, et al. Physical activity in relation to knee cartilage T2 progression measured with 3 T MRI over a period of 1 years: data from the Osteoarthritis Initiative. Osteoarthritis Cartilage 2013;21(10):1558–66.

30. Welsch GH, Apprich S, Zbyn S, et al. Biochemical (T2, T2* and magnetisation transfer ratio) MRI of knee cartilage: feasibility at ultra-high field (7T) compared with high field (3T) strength. Eur Radiol 2011;21(6):1136–43.

31. Lazik A, Theysohn JM, Geis C, et al. 7 Tesla quantitative hip MRI: T1, T2 and T2* mapping of hip cartilage in healthy volunteers. Eur Radiol 2016;26(5): 1245–53.

32. Domayer SE, Apprich S, Stelzeneder D, et al. Cartilage repair of the ankle: first results of T2 mapping at 7.0 T after microfracture and matrix associated autologous cartilage transplantation. Osteoarthritis Cartilage 2012;20(8):829–36.

33. Chang G, Xia D, Sherman O, et al. High resolution morphologic imaging and T2 mapping of cartilage

at 7 Tesla: comparison of cartilage repair patients and healthy controls. MAGMA 2013;26(6):539–48.

34. Heule R, Bar P, Mirkes C, et al. Triple-echo steady-state T2 relaxometry of the human brain at high to ultra-high fields. NMR Biomed 2014;27(9):1037–45.

35. Heule R, Ganter C, Bieri O. Triple echo steady-state (TESS) relaxometry. Magn Reson Med 2014;71(1):230–7.

36. Juras V, Zbyn S, Mlynarik V, et al. The compositional difference between ankle and knee cartilage demonstrated by T2 mapping at 7 Tesla MR. Eur J Radiol 2016;85(4):771–7.

37. Kraff O, Lazik-Palm A, Heule R, et al. 7 Tesla quantitative hip MRI: a comparison between TESS and CPMG for T2 mapping. MAGMA 2016;29(3):503–12.

38. Juras V, Schreiner M, Laurent D, et al. The comparison of the performance of 3T and 7T T2 mapping for untreated low-grade cartilage lesions. Magn Reson Imaging 2019;55:86–92.

39. Pauly JM, Conolly SI, Nishimura DG, et al. Slice-selective excitation for very short T2 species. Proc 8th Annual Meeting ISMRM; 1989; Amsterdam; 1989. p. Abstract 28.

40. Du J, Bydder M, Takahashi AM, et al. Two-dimensional ultrashort echo time imaging using a spiral trajectory. Magn Reson Imaging 2008;26(3):304–12.

41. Rahmer J, Bornert P, Groen J, et al. Three-dimensional radial ultrashort echo-time imaging with T2 adapted sampling. Magn Reson Med 2006;55(5):1075–82.

42. Grodzki DM, Jakob PM, Heismann B. Ultrashort echo time imaging using pointwise encoding time reduction with radial acquisition (PETRA). Magn Reson Med 2012;67(2):510–8.

43. Krug R, Larson PE, Wang C, et al. Ultrashort echo time MRI of cortical bone at 7 tesla field strength: a feasibility study. J Magn Reson Imaging 2011;34(3):691–5.

44. Juras V, Zbyn S, Pressl C, et al. Regional variations of T(2)* in healthy and pathologic achilles tendon in vivo at 7 Tesla: preliminary results. Magn Reson Med 2012;68(5):1607–13.

45. Larson PE, Han M, Krug R, et al. Ultrashort echo time and zero echo time MRI at 7T. MAGMA 2016;29(3):359–70.

46. Sepponen RE, Pohjonen JA, Sipponen JT, et al. A method for T1 rho imaging. J Comput Assist Tomogr 1985;9(6):1007–11.

47. Gilani IA, Sepponen R. Quantitative rotating frame relaxometry methods in MRI. NMR Biomed 2016;29(6):841–61.

48. Keenan KE, Besier TF, Pauly JM, et al. Prediction of glycosaminoglycan content in human cartilage by age, T1rho and T2 MRI. Osteoarthritis Cartilage 2011;19(2):171–9.

49. Wang L, Chang G, Xu J, et al. T1rho MRI of menisci and cartilage in patients with osteoarthritis at 3T. Eur J Radiol 2012;81(9):2329–36.

50. Sharafi A, Xia D, Chang G, et al. Biexponential T1rho relaxation mapping of human knee cartilage in vivo at 3 T. NMR Biomed 2017;30(10).

51. Singh A, Haris M, Cai K, et al. High resolution T1rho mapping of in vivo human knee cartilage at 7T. PLoS One 2014;9(5):e97486.

52. Wyatt C, Guha A, Venkatachari A, et al. Improved differentiation between knees with cartilage lesions and controls using 7T relaxation time mapping. J Orthop Translat 2015;3(4):197–204.

53. Ling W, Regatte RR, Navon G, et al. Assessment of glycosaminoglycan concentration in vivo by chemical exchange-dependent saturation transfer (gagCEST). Proc Natl Acad Sci U S A 2008;105(7):2266–70.

54. Schmitt B, Zbyn S, Stelzeneder D, et al. Cartilage quality assessment by using glycosaminoglycan chemical exchange saturation transfer and (23)Na MR imaging at 7 T. Radiology 2011;260(1):257–64.

55. Singh A, Haris M, Cai K, et al. Chemical exchange saturation transfer magnetic resonance imaging of human knee cartilage at 3 T and 7 T. Magn Reson Med 2012;68(2):588–94.

56. Haris M, Singh A, Reddy S, et al. Characterization of viscosupplementation formulations using chemical exchange saturation transfer (ViscoCEST). J Transl Med 2016;14:92.

57. Krishnamoorthy G, Nanga RPR, Bagga P, et al. High quality three-dimensional gagCEST imaging of in vivo human knee cartilage at 7 Tesla. Magn Reson Med 2017;77(5):1866–73.

58. Kogan F, Hargreaves BA, Gold GE. Volumetric multi-slice gagCEST imaging of articular cartilage: Optimization and comparison with T1rho. Magn Reson Med 2017;77(3):1134–41.

59. Brinkhof S, Nizak R, Khlebnikov V, et al. Detection of early cartilage damage: feasibility and potential of gagCEST imaging at 7T. Eur Radiol 2018;28(7):2874–81.

60. Madelin G, Lee JS, Regatte RR, et al. Sodium MRI: methods and applications. Prog Nucl Magn Reson Spectrosc 2014;79:14–47.

61. Moon CH, Kim JH, Zhao T, et al. Quantitative (23) Na MRI of human knee cartilage using dual-tuned (1) H/(23) Na transceiver array radiofrequency coil at 7 tesla. J Magn Reson Imaging 2013;38(5):1063–72.

62. Wiggins GC, Brown R, Lakshmanan K. High-performance radiofrequency coils for (23)Na MRI: brain and musculoskeletal applications. NMR Biomed 2016;29(2):96–106.

63. Pipe JG, Zwart NR, Aboussouan EA, et al. A new design and rationale for 3D orthogonally over-sampled k-space trajectories. Magn Reson Med 2011;66(5):1303–11.

64. Nagel AM, Laun FB, Weber MA, et al. Sodium MRI using a density-adapted 3D radial acquisition technique. Magn Reson Med 2009;62(6):1565–73.

65. Gurney PT, Hargreaves BA, Nishimura DG. Design and analysis of a practical 3D cones trajectory. Magn Reson Med 2006;55(3):575–82.

66. Idiyatullin D, Corum C, Park JY, et al. Fast and quiet MRI using a swept radiofrequency. J Magn Reson 2006;181(2):342–9.

67. Weiger M, Pruessmann KP, Hennel F. MRI with zero echo time: hard versus sweep pulse excitation. Magn Reson Med 2011;66(2):379–89.

68. Madelin G, Chang G, Otazo R, et al. Compressed sensing sodium MRI of cartilage at 7T: preliminary study. J Magn Reson 2012;214(1):360–5.

69. Wheaton AJ, Borthakur A, Shapiro EM, et al. Proteoglycan loss in human knee cartilage: quantitation with sodium MR imaging–feasibility study. Radiology 2004;231(3):900–5.

70. Chang G, Madelin G, Sherman OH, et al. Improved assessment of cartilage repair tissue using fluid-suppressed (2)(3)Na inversion recovery MRI at 7 Tesla: preliminary results. Eur Radiol 2012;22(6): 1341–9.

71. Madelin G, Babb J, Xia D, et al. Articular cartilage: evaluation with fluid-suppressed 7.0-T sodium MR imaging in subjects with and subjects without osteoarthritis. Radiology 2013;268(2):481–91.

72. Clausen T. Na+-K+ pump regulation and skeletal muscle contractility. Physiol Rev 2003;83(4): 1269–324.

73. Chang G, Wang L, Schweitzer ME, et al. 3D 23Na MRI of human skeletal muscle at 7 Tesla: initial experience. Eur Radiol 2010;20(8):2039–46.

74. Amarteifio E, Nagel AM, Weber MA, et al. Hyperkalemic periodic paralysis and permanent weakness: 3-T MR imaging depicts intracellular 23Na overload–initial results. Radiology 2012;264(1):154–63.

75. Kopp C, Linz P, Dahlmann A, et al. 23Na magnetic resonance imaging-determined tissue sodium in healthy subjects and hypertensive patients. Hypertension 2013;61(3):635–40.

76. Chance B, Eleff S, Leigh JS Jr, et al. Mitochondrial regulation of phosphocreatine/inorganic phosphate ratios in exercising human muscle: a gated 31P NMR study. Proc Natl Acad Sci U S A 1981;78(11): 6714–8.

77. Kemp GJ, Radda GK. Quantitative interpretation of bioenergetic data from 31P and 1H magnetic resonance spectroscopic studies of skeletal muscle: an analytical review. Magn Reson Q 1994;10(1): 43–63.

78. Kuhl CK, Layer G, Traber F, et al. Mitochondrial encephalomyopathy: correlation of P-31 exercise MR spectroscopy with clinical findings. Radiology 1994;192(1):223–30.

79. Taylor DJ. Clinical utility of muscle MR spectroscopy. Semin Musculoskelet Radiol 2000;4(4):481–502.

80. Scheuermann-Freestone M, Madsen PL, Manners D, et al. Abnormal cardiac and skeletal muscle energy metabolism in patients with type 2 diabetes. Circulation 2003;107(24):3040–6.

81. Schunk K, Romaneehsen B, Rieker O, et al. Dynamic phosphorus-31 magnetic resonance spectroscopy in arterial occlusive disease: effects of vascular therapy on spectroscopic results. Invest Radiol 1998;33(6):329–35.

82. McCully KK, Argov Z, Boden BP, et al. Detection of muscle injury in humans with 31-P magnetic resonance spectroscopy. Muscle Nerve 1988;11(3): 212–6.

83. Bogner W, Chmelik M, Schmid AI, et al. Assessment of (31)P relaxation times in the human calf muscle: a comparison between 3 T and 7 T in vivo. Magn Reson Med 2009;62(3):574–82.

84. Parasoglou P, Feng L, Xia D, et al. Rapid 3D-imaging of phosphocreatine recovery kinetics in the human lower leg muscles with compressed sensing. Magn Reson Med 2012;68(6):1738–46.

85. Parasoglou P, Xia D, Chang G, et al. Dynamic three-dimensional imaging of phosphocreatine recovery kinetics in the human lower leg muscles at 3T and 7T: a preliminary study. NMR Biomed 2013;26(3): 348–56.

86. Hooijmans MT, Doorenweerd N, Baligand C, et al. Spatially localized phosphorous metabolism of skeletal muscle in Duchenne muscular dystrophy patients: 24-month follow-up. PLoS One 2017;12(8): e0182086.

87. Korzowski A, Bachert P. High-resolution (31 P echo-planar spectroscopic imaging in vivo at 7T. Magn Reson Med 2018;79(3):1251–9.

88. Schmid AI, Meyerspeer M, Robinson SD, et al. Dynamic PCr and pH imaging of human calf muscles during exercise and recovery using (31) P gradient-Echo MRI at 7 Tesla. Magn Reson Med 2016;75(6):2324–31.

Printed and bound by CPI Group (UK) Ltd, Croydon, CR0 4YY

08/05/2025

01864692-0009